The Reference Shelf®

U.S. National Debate Topic 2007–2008

Health Care in Sub-Saharan Africa

Edited by Forrest Cole

Editorial Advisor Lynn M. Messina

The Reference Shelf
Volume 79 • Number 3

The H. W. Wilson Company
2007

The Reference Shelf

The books in this series contain reprints of articles, excerpts from books, addresses on current issues, and studies of social trends in the United States and other countries. There are six separately bound numbers in each volume, all of which are usually published in the same calendar year. Numbers one through five are each devoted to a single subject, providing background information and discussion from various points of view and concluding with a subject index and comprehensive bibliography that lists books, pamphlets, and abstracts of additional articles on the subject. The final number of each volume is a collection of recent speeches, and it contains a cumulative speaker index. Books in the series may be purchased individually or on subscription.

Library of Congress has cataloged this serial title as follows:

U.S. national debate topic 2007-2008 : health care in Sub-Saharan Africa / edited by Forrest Cole; editorial advisor, Lynn M. Messina.
    p. cm. — (The reference shelf ; v. 79, no. 3)
    ISBN 978-0-8242-1069-4 (alk. paper)
    1. Medical care—Africa, Sub-Saharan. I. Cole, Forrest. II. Title: Health care in Sub-Saharan Africa.
        RA395.A5548U86 2007
        362.10967—dc22

                                                            2007011925

Cover: A doctor treats a child at Benedir Hospital in Mogadishu, Somalia, on March 9, 2007. (STRINGER/AFP/Getty Images)

Visit H. W. Wilson's Web site: www.hwwilson.com

Printed in the United States of America

Contents

Preface

History is replete with stories of European colonizers attempting to "civilize" nations and societies they considered less developed than their own. Those European countries that participated in the "Scramble for Africa" in the 19th century had a profound and not always positive effect on the continent. Over the course of nearly 100 years, virtually every country in Africa was colonized, and as the Europeans attempted to transform the tribal cultures into societies more closely resembling those in the West, the way Africans lived changed immensely. This was especially true in the geographically immense area of sub-Saharan Africa, defined by its location south of the Sahara Desert and by its ethnic, cultural, and political differences from North Africa. Unfortunately, once these sub-Saharan countries began to achieve their independence after World War II, they were virtually abandoned by the international community and left without the proper structures to continue life as it had been. A return to traditional culture at this point was impossible, and governing and caring for themselves under the foreign structures imposed by Europeans made for a difficult transition.

One of the most affected areas of African society was the health care system. During the colonial period, cultures that had once depended on traditional healers like the *Sangomas* of South Africa were placed under the care of the church and state. However, as these countries gained their independence, it became necessary to instill a more relative system that varied according to each culture. This process could not be completed overnight, and consequently a resurgence of disease resulted due to lack of education, deficient health care systems, and cultural taboos that interfered with procuring proper care.

HIV/AIDS has been one of the most devastating diseases to affect sub-Saharan Africa. Although most of the early cases were detected in the United States, scientists have since suggested that the first documented case of AIDS was likely identified in the Congo in the late 1950s. In the past 15 years, HIV/AIDS infections have skyrocketed in Africa. At one point, it was reported that as many as one in four South Africans were afflicted with the disease. Chapter 1 presents a variety of articles that discuss the current AIDS situation and its possible remedies in sub-Saharan Africa. An area that has drawn particular concern, discussed in Chapter 2, is the increasing prevalence of HIV/AIDS in women and children. Due to the social constructs of certain African cultures, men may have multiple sex partners, and it is not only taboo for a man to wear protection, but it is also considered disrespectful for a woman to suggest it. The articles selected propose possible strategies to change the way women are treated domestically and medically, given the great concern not only for their well-being, but also for their children's. Indeed, the number of AIDS orphans has been growing exponentially each year, and while most of these children do not contract the disease themselves, they are often left without care and support.

Though the HIV/AIDS pandemic has garnered mass attention in and out of Africa, researchers, scientists, health care providers, and some philanthropists are attempting to ensure that people do not overlook what have been termed "neglected diseases." Chapter 3 features articles that discuss the various problems encountered in combating tuberculosis, malaria, and other tropical diseases, as well as their possible solutions. Chapter 4 presents specific difficulties and some of the various methods that have been suggested to improve the health care system in sub-Saharan Africa, including importing health care workers from elsewhere in Africa, creating relationships between private and public health care institutions, using traditional cures, and focusing on regional support.

Finally, as sub-Saharan Africa has reached a state of crisis, Chapter 5 looks at the issue of U.S. aid to the region. Most of the articles focus on the HIV/AIDS pandemic because of President Bush's PEPFAR campaign to combat the disease internationally, but sub-Saharan Africa has become the topic of the moment, and more and more aid is being supplied via programs initiated by the United States. The question now is whether or not that aid will be enough.

I would like to extend my gratitude to all the authors and publications that have granted permission to reprint their work in this collection. Also, I would like to especially thank Lynn M. Messina, Richard Stein, Paul McCaffrey, David Ramm, Ronald Eniclerico, and Christopher Mari for their help and advice with this project.

Forrest Cole
June 2007

I. THE HIV/AIDS PANDEMIC

HIV/AIDS: THE TREATMENT GAP

Estimated worldwide coverage with antiretroviral treatment, end 2003

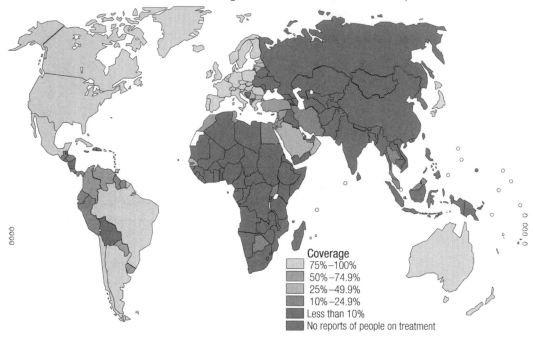

Coverage
- 75%–100%
- 50%–74.9%
- 25%–49.9%
- 10%–24.9%
- Less than 10%
- No reports of people on treatment

HIV/AIDS: 3 BY 5 INITIATIVE

Countries that have requested assistance under the 3 by 5 initiative, as of 3 March 2004

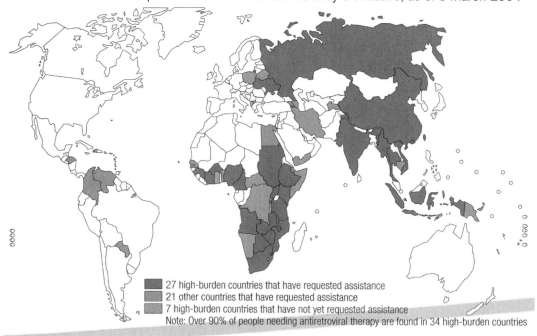

- 27 high-burden countries that have requested assistance
- 21 other countries that have requested assistance
- 7 high-burden countries that have not yet requested assistance

Note: Over 90% of people needing antiretroviral therapy are found in 34 high-burden countries

Editor's Introduction

In 2006 the United Nations reported that an estimated 24.5 million people were living with HIV/AIDS in sub-Saharan Africa, and that during 2005 alone over 2 million Africans died from the disease. These figures are staggering, especially when one considers that they are likely incomplete. Indeed, cultural taboos and limited access to rural or otherwise secluded locales virtually assures that AIDS deaths are underreported. Though the availability of education, HIV counseling, and health care, particularly antiretroviral drugs (ARVs), is steadily increasing, the number of infections continues to rise at a meteoric rate. While some countries, such as Uganda, have managed to stabilize their infection rates, the rates in other nations, particularly in the south, have risen to as high as 30 percent of the population.

Given such realities, the continent's HIV/AIDS problem cannot be solved by Africans alone. Nevertheless, international assistance has not yet proven a decisive factor in the struggle. While Africa has received a great influx of foreign aid over the past decade, cultural and economic factors, as well as ineffective distribution networks and coordination disparities, have impeded progress. In the first article in this chapter, "HIV/AIDS Care in Africa Today," Allan R. Ronald and Merle A. Sande focus on strategies to implement that could counteract the AIDS epidemic. They call for the worldwide promotion of HIV education, special consideration for those already afflicted with the disease, and encouragement of other countries to follow the example of Uganda, which reversed the devastation dramatically. Among the methods they propose are a wider use of public/private partnerships, education initiatives aimed at countering cultural taboos, and a call for a larger commitment from local and global leadership.

In the next article, "The African AIDS Crisis and International Indifference," Mpho Selemogo, a recent medical school graduate, presents striking statistics about the number of people living in poverty in sub-Saharan Africa and how this directly impacts their ability to learn about the effects and proper treatment of HIV. He discusses both sides of the argument concerning whether wealthier nations are obligated to help developing countries through the crisis and points out that, despite considerable aid from certain quarters, often the delivered amounts fall short of targets. According to Selemogo, this shortfall becomes problematic for organizations whose treatment plans depend on receiving the full allotment of promised aid.

The influence of the church is another major factor in the fight against the spread of HIV/AIDS. With over 130 million Roman Catholics in Africa, the Vatican holds considerable sway in the region. However, although there is ample proof that condom use helps prevent the spread of HIV and thus saves lives, the Church has stood firmly behind its 1968 encyclical *Humanae Vitae*, which holds that condoms "thwart conception" and are thus antithetical to Christian morality. Nevertheless, as Marcella Alsan notes, in "The Church & AIDS in Africa," 25 percent of the care administered to African AIDS victims is provided by Catholic organizations. Moreover, many in the Church, including high-ranking African clergy, have concluded that the "preservation of human life is paramount" and supersedes concerns about the morality of condom use. Still, Alsan believes that the Vatican misunderstands current widespread gender inequalities in sub-Saharan Africa, citing the prevalence of teenage brides, many of whom contract the HIV virus from their typically older husbands who were most likely infected prior to marriage.

In the fourth article, "To Tackle Taboo: How Africa Is Opening up a New Front in the Fight Against AIDS," Andrew Jack discusses how certain African cultural practices foster inequality between men and women and promote the spread of the HIV virus. Particularly, he singles out traditional polygamy, which encourages men to have multiple sex partners and contributes to higher infection rates among women. Though some critics claim that such notions are rooted in western stereotypes of African men, statistics largely support Jack's analysis. To counteract these harmful patterns, Jack proposes that Africans be educated as to the benefits of having fewer sex partners, and that prevention, rather than treatment, be the focus of anti-HIV/AIDs initiatives.

The final piece in this chapter, "Giving Away HIV Drugs Is Not as Easy as It Seems," published by AIDS Alert, shows that despite efforts by some pharmaceutical companies to increase the availability of ARVs by reducing their cost or providing them free of charge, distributing these drugs to patients has proven supremely difficult. The chief impediment has been incomplete or nonexistent health care infrastructure. Many of these companies are now joining with non-profits and NGOs to construct better distribution networks, but much more work remains to be done.

HIV/AIDS Care in Africa Today

By Allan R. Ronald and Merle A. Sande
Clinical Infectious Diseases, April 1, 2005

Light is appearing at the end of the proverbial tunnel throughout the regions of sub-Saharan Africa that are currently being decimated by AIDS. A remarkable congruence of 3 major streams of endeavor portends the success of our shared efforts to limit the ravages of HIV infection and begin winning the war against AIDS on several fronts. The first endeavor is to ensure that the incredible, indescribable plight of individuals dying of AIDS is being heard by individuals, organizations, and governments around the world. AIDS-associated tragedies, such as the 8000 deaths that occur each day, the fact that a new child is orphaned every 14 years, and the collapsing of economies, have raised the topic of AIDS to the forefront of the global conscience [1]. As a result, the world is rolling up its sleeves and is beginning to respond [2]. The "3 by 5" initiatives of the World Health Organization have set forth the goal that 3 million HIV-infected individuals in developing countries will be receiving antiretroviral treatment by 31 December 2005. A second endeavor is the opportunity to make a difference for sick, frequently impoverished patients with AIDS who are awaiting death. Although, in the West, we have only prescribed antiretrovirals effectively since 1996, we already know that the vast majority of HIV-infected individuals—presumably, almost 90% of such individuals—can remain well and can fulfill their desires and responsibilities within the home, workplace, and community for at least 5 years thanks to these complex but life-sustaining regimens [3]. The world has found multiple ways to bring the cost of antiretrovirals into a reasonable price range. Finally, a third endeavor, which is equally important but is readily forgotten, is the success story that has unfolded in Uganda, where the prevalence and incidence of HIV infection have been dramatically reduced [4]. This endeavor provides hope that, collectively, individuals and societies can change behaviors, reduce risks, and alter transmission dynamics so that, even in the absence of an AIDS vaccine, marked reductions in the global incidence of HIV infection will occur within the next 5 years.

In their report, Wester et al. [5] summarized the lessons that they have learned from their experiences with the antiretroviral treatment clinic established through the auspices of the Botswana–Harvard School of Public Health AIDS Initiative Partnership for HIV

Research and Education in Gaborone, Botswana. They also reported an important innovation in the fight against HIV/AIDS in Africa: the public-private partnership (in this case, a partnership involving The Merck Company Foundation/Merck & Company, the Bill & Melinda Gates Foundation, Harvard University, and the government of Botswana. The lessons learned from their experiences, our own experiences, and experiences at sites elsewhere in sub-Saharan Africa need to be assimilated, and dozens of sites for HIV/AIDS care need to developed, with the goal of achieving the 3 by 5 targets of the World Health Organization through the cooperative efforts and largess of the global society.

The Academic Alliance for AIDS Care and Prevention in Africa Foundation (see the Academic Alliance Foundation Web site, which is available at http://www.academicalliancefoundation.org/) is a similar public-private partnership that was created in 2000 as a partnership between Ugandan and North American physicians in academic medicine, Pfizer Pharmaceuticals and the Pfizer Foundation, and the Makerere University Faculty of Medicine and Mulago Hospital in Kampala, Uganda. With a firm handshake and the blessing of Ugandan President Yoweri Musevani, the Uganda Ministry of Health, and the Uganda AIDS Commission, the consortium began to build its programs in June 2001. In early 2002, expanded clinics were opened, and a 4-week physician-training course was organized and taught in partnership and cooperation with trainers from the Infectious Diseases Society of America. Our experiences were similar to those in Botswana. Our limited facilities at Mulago Hospital (the large national referral hospital in Kampala, which faces staffing and crowding problems similar to those noted at Princess Marina Hospital in Gaborone, as well as an HIV seroprevalence rate of 65% among the medical wards) were quickly overwhelmed, and sick patients who required care appeared from everywhere. Most patients were poor, and many were illiterate. Within 3 years, >8000 HIV-infected individuals have been registered in our adult and pediatric clinics. Fortunately, in 2003, we were awarded a pilot grant from the Bill & Melinda Gates Foundation and were able to (1) initiate studies of HIV prevention in the era of increased access to antiretrovirals and (2) perform operational research in the clinic setting. Now, 3 years after the opening of the expanded clinics, what has been achieved? What might we have done differently?

We were fortunate to work within a society that has created a substantial infrastructure for the prevention of HIV infection, albeit an infrastructure that is less developed for the treatment and care of patients with HIV infection. The prevalence of HIV infection has decreased by >50% during the past 12 years; this decrease in prevalence has been accompanied by a decrease in the incidence of HIV infection, particularly among patients in younger age groups (i.e., patients <20 years of age) [5]. Expanded access to care ideally should occur in a setting in which prevention is a primary priority of both the government and the organizations responsible for program delivery. The reasons underlying the success achieved in Uganda are still being debated, but they include inspired presidential leadership; emphasis on the "ABC's" (i.e., **A**bstinence, **B**e faithful [or "zero grazing"], and **C**ondom access for risky behaviors); processes that facilitated the emergence of >2000 nongovernmental organizations, including initiatives by religious organizations; limited controversy with regard to promotion of condom use; and reduced stigma because of societal acceptance of HIV infection as a diagnosis and of AIDS as a cause of death. Other countries, presumably including Botswana, are also expanding programs that will reduce the incidence of HIV infection. As the world and its institutions focus on HIV/AIDS care, prevention must be emphasized and must remain a primary objective [6].

Now we need a sustained commitment from leadership to provide enhanced care for individual patients with AIDS, including access to antiretroviral treatment. Few countries have made significant revisions of their national budgets or, even, their national priorities to address issues of care. In societies devastated by AIDS, there has

---

As the world and its institutions focus on HIV/AIDS care, prevention must be emphasized and must remain a primary objective.

---

been little serious preparation by most governments, universities, or health care institutions to prepare to meet the massive human and fiscal resources required to provide even limited programs of HIV/AIDS care. Despite the eloquent arguments of Nelson Mandela, Stephen Lewis, Bill Clinton, and others, antiretroviral treatment for HIV-infected individuals has received token support from national leaders in Africa. This must change.

Fiscal resources are often cited as the primary problem associated with the rapid expansion of care programs. Although this is "politically correct," in 2004, finances in most countries were not a primary obstacle to providing "enhanced care." Monies that are made available (through The Global Fund for AIDS, Tuberculosis, and Malaria; The World Bank; The President's Emergency Plan for AIDS Relief, etc.) often are not spent efficiently within expected time frames, because of the lack of visionary leadership, inadequate human resources, poorly developed business plans, or multitiered bureaucracy. This has occurred even in Uganda, despite its forward-looking government. In a sincere effort to avoid misallocation of funds, most countries have established criteria and processes that are a challenge to navigate efficiently. As a result, the introduction of expanded, scaled-up care programs takes years, instead of months, to accomplish. "Business as usual" will not suffice if we wish to take advantage of the billions of monies available to provide HIV/AIDS care and reduce by 50% the number of deaths due to

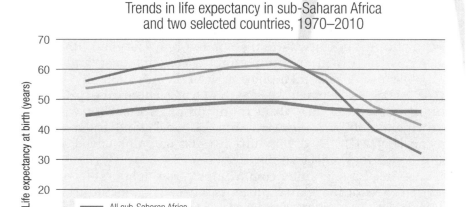

THE IMPACT OF HIV/AIDS IN AFRICA

Trends in life expectancy in sub-Saharan Africa
and two selected countries, 1970–2010

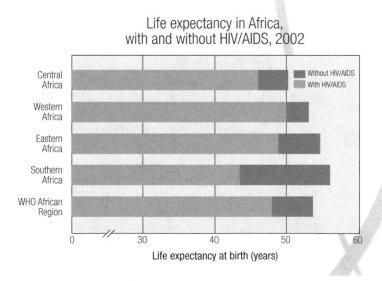

Life expectancy in Africa,
with and without HIV/AIDS, 2002

The United Nations is the author of the original material.

AIDS that will otherwise occur between now and 2010. Organizational structures must be renewed, and there must be a sustained, serious commitment of national and institutional leadership to rapidly deploy both the human and fiscal resources necessary for this massive public undertaking. Care and prevention organizations that demonstrate effective and efficient financial structures, as well as accountability, must be rewarded with available resources that can be deployed to patient care quickly and effectively.

In Botswana, Wester et al. [5] also identified the need to build treatment capacity with additional trained human resources. At our site, we have trained 300 physicians to train other physicians to become trainers themselves, including 68 physicians from 13 African countries outside Uganda. These individuals have been tasked and have been given the skill set to provide training when they return to their own environment. Although monitoring/evaluation processes are only now in place to critically assess the effectiveness of the training program, we sense that most of the trainees have the capacity to deliver competent HIV/AIDS care.

The challenges associated with providing HIV/AIDS care are immense. Many HIV-infected patients present with a serious AIDS-defining illness, and the mortality rate associated with this initial illness approaches 50%. In most African countries, the public resources available for the care of patients with such life-threatening serious infections as cryptococcal meningitis, advanced tuberculosis, or *Toxoplasma* encephalitis are limited and are frequently nonexistent. Large numbers of patients die because they receive inadequate care during their initial illness. Widespread voluntary counseling and testing is one response that will enable HIV-positive individuals to enter care programs before the occurrence of an end-of-life scenario and, also, to reduce their likelihood of infecting other individuals. Tragically, <10% of HIV-infected Africans know their HIV infection status. We have introduced voluntary counseling and testing into the medical wards of Mulago Hospital, where the prevalence of HIV infection is >65%, and we have found that (1) most patients accept testing when it is offered freely, and (2) they are prepared to enter care programs. With the support of external funding from the Bill & Melinda Gates Foundation, we have been able to demonstrate the acceptability of voluntary counseling and testing, and, with the use of funds from the President's Emergency Plan for AIDS Relief, such services are being widely implemented in Uganda.

Other impediments to widespread access to antiretroviral treatment exist. What is the minimum number of laboratory tests needed to ensure adequate care? How can these tests be effectively, efficiently, and inexpensively performed—particularly in rural areas, where most individuals reside? New strategies and markedly reduced costs for tests, including CD4 cell counts and viral load determinations, are being developed. Drug logistics have to be efficient, and the supply chain has to work all the time, or treatment failure will rapidly occur. Governments in many parts of Africa have a deplorable record of ensuring an adequate supply of drugs and diagnostics, even when the drugs and diagnostics are freely supplied. Perhaps the private sector, which can adequately ensure access to a cold, carbonated, nonalcoholic beverage at thousands of locations in Uganda, can also ensure that drugs arrive at the point of care. Bold new approaches are needed. Systems experts who can provide advice and training to ensure the creation of new and efficient public-private partnerships that enable the delivery of services are essential. A new vertical HIV service is not sustainable and will only divert resources from a health care system that is in desperate need of support.

Adequate adherence to antiretroviral treatment has been presumed to be difficult to achieve within Africa. Fortunately, all studies that have appeared to date have suggested that, with appropriate training, motivation, and supervision, adherence will be possible [7]. This does not imply that adherence will be "easy" to achieve. Although HIV prevention must remain the first priority of all of us who are working in the field of HIV/AIDS care, prevention of the development of resistance among HIV isolates is a close second within Africa. We have demonstrated that, in our patients in Kampala, the development of resistance among HIV isolates is most likely to occur in patients who miss drug doses for >2 days. Close monitoring and counseling regarding the use of antiretrovirals must ensure that these "drug holidays" are minimized. Drug-resistant HIV isolates not only result in the failure of drug therapy for the infected individual, but these resistant strains can also be transmitted to other individuals, rendering the use of first-line regimens ineffective for the newly infected patient. It is our hope that the median time to clinical failure of first-line regimens will be at least 5 years, if not longer. This will ensure that most individuals will not require second- and third-line therapies within the next 5 years and thereby frustrate efforts to roll out first-line regimens to millions of individuals.

> The urgent need for operational research to aid in the direction of "care programs" cannot be overemphasized.

The urgent need for operational research to aid in the direction of "care programs" cannot be overemphasized. We have initiated prospective studies of HIV-associated complications, such as visual impairment, hepatic disease, neurological infections, dementia, Kaposi sarcoma, and other complications that arise from the epidemic, and we have developed simple, affordable interventions that hopefully can enhance care in the rural and urban environments. Although research is essential to enable HIV/AIDS care in Africa, widespread access to care cannot await the results of research. Research and HIV/AIDS care must proceed in parallel, and, in this case, "the boat must be built as it sails from the harbor."

Finally, public-private partnerships (such as the program in Botswana discussed in the report by Wester et al. [5] and our own Academic Alliance Program in Uganda) have the potential to make enormous contributions to the fight against HIV/AIDS in Africa and elsewhere. However, as we work together to create and scale up care and prevention programs, it is essential to monitor and evaluate the effectiveness of such programs. Donors, including the US Government, as well as the governments of host countries, should insist on documentation of the results of their investments and evidence of the effective use of antiretroviral drugs, including measures of adherence, prevention of resistance, and management of side effects, as well as implementation of prevention initiatives and sustainability of productive lives. Only programs that can achieve those goals and document the results should continue to be eligible for funding.

In summary, many lessons can be learned from the experiences of the alliances that are being formed between HIV caregivers in Africa and in Western countries. To paraphrase Winston Churchill during the early days of World War II, "We have not reached the beginning of the end, but perhaps we are approaching the end of the beginning."

References

1. Hogg R, Cahn P, Katabira E, Lange J. Time to act: global apathy towards HIV/AIDS is a crime against humanity. Lancet **2002**; 360:1710–1.

2. World Health Organization (WHO)/Joint United Nations Programme on HIV/AIDS (UNAIDS). Treating 3 million by 2005: making it happen. The WHO strategy. France: WHO/AIDS, 2003.
   Available at: http://www.who.int/3by5/publications/documents/isbn9241591129/en/.
   Accessed 23 February **2005**.

3. Egger M, May M, Chene G, et al. Prognosis of HIV-1-infected patients starting highly active antiretroviral therapy: a collaborative analysis of prospective studies. ART Cohort Collaboration. Lancet **2002**; 360:119–29.

4. Stoneburner RL, Low-Beer D. Population-level HIV declines and behavioral risk avoidance in Uganda. Science 2004; 304:714–8.

5. Wester CW, Bussmann H, Avalos A, et al. Establishment of a public antiretroviral treatment clinic for adults in urban Botswana: lessons learned. Clin Infect Dis **2005**; 40:1041–4 (in this issue).

6. Gayle HD. Curbing the global AIDS epidemic. N Engl J Med **2003**; 348:1802–5.

7. Oyugi JH, Byakika-Tusiime J, Charlebois ED, et al. Multiple validated measures of adherence indicate high levels of adherence to generic HIV antiretroviral therapy in a resource-limited setting. J Acquir Immune Defic Syndr **2004**; 36:1100–2.

The African AIDS Crisis and International Indifference

BY MPHO SELEMOGO
THE HUMANIST, JANUARY/FEBRUARY 2006

I have never been to Africa. I am not black. I do not have HIV. . . . By virtue of my work, I have cared for people—transiently—who have HIV/AIDS. But, as politically incorrect as it may sound, I am not connected to the tragedy that is AIDS in Africa. And, as crass as it may sound, I do not have to be. Perhaps, as part of my effort to be reasonably well-informed about the world, I cannot avoid hearing about it. . . . But I can avoid doing anything about it, and no one will call me to account for my inaction. . . . Tragedy is not an easily exported commodity, and we prefer that it be handled behind national borders. In wealthier nations, we look after our own.

These words by Joel Pauls Wohlgemut, appearing in his 2002 prize-winning Canadian Medical Association Journal article, "AIDS, Africa and indifference: A confession," are arguably some of the most courageous to appear in the academic literature in recent times. It is a confession of indifference: indifference to the African AIDS crisis that now claims the lives of about 5,000 Africans daily and accounts for 80 percent of the world's AIDS deaths. Africa is also a continent that houses 95 percent of the world's AIDS orphans, 70 percent of the people newly infected by HIV, and 90 percent of the world's children living with HIV/AIDS. Needless to say, the amount of human suffering behind these figures is almost unimaginable. "Viewed from the perspective of suffering," writes P. Farmer and A. Kleinman in "AIDS as Human Suffering" (published in 1998 in P. J. Brown's *Understanding and Applying Medical Anthropology*), AIDS must rank with smallpox, plague, and leprosy in its capacity to menace and hurt, to burden and spoil human experience, and to elicit questions about the nature of life and its significance. Suffering extends from those inflicted . . . to their families and intimates, to the practitioners and institutions who care for them, and to their neighborhoods and the rest of society.

Africa's past advances in human development have been literally reversed by the HIV/AIDS epidemic, with indices such as life expectancy plummeting by twenty years in some countries. The burden of this pandemic no doubt presents an economic nightmare for an economy already in distress—where about 300 million (approximately 50 percent) of the continent's people live in extreme poverty, fewer than half the children complete primary school, and drought cycles have become more frequent, greatly affecting the capacity to produce food. Recently, proportions of the African population having access to health services, safe water, and sanitation have been reported to be 51 percent, 40 percent, and 31 percent, respectively. The debt burden for Africa stood at

> Most African countries are just too poor to doctor themselves against AIDS and its consequences.

$315 billion in 2000, and all African countries except the Republic of South Africa were reported to be spending more on servicing this debt than on health care. With some African countries now receiving aid in the form of loans, the economic situation can only get worse.

Accounting for less than 1 percent of world exports, it is clear that Africa will never emerge from the AIDS calamity on its own. Despite aspirations of better healthcare for all Africans, many would now agree that most African countries are just too poor to doctor themselves against AIDS and its consequences. Perhaps what remains their only hope is that other nations, acting out of concern and respect for human dignity or whatever moral code, might come to their aid and provide relief.

Over the past years, however, the AIDS crisis in Africa has worsened to catastrophic levels, with little being done to arrest the progress of the disease there because many in the affluent world, as A. Trowbridge wrote in the November/December 2000 *Humanist,* "looked upon assistance to Africa as charity that they had a right to offer or withhold." As a consequence, with too few domestic resources of its own, what contributions Africa has received have had little meaningful success in staunching the growth of HIV and AIDS on that continent. The 1990s saw the commitments of many donors decline to a trickle and become increasingly sporadic. Aid levels have dropped relative to the growth of HIV—to the extent that the lack of finances has become the primary constraint on progress against AIDS in Africa. And as we saw recently when the G-8 met at Gleneagles in Scotland, it now takes the world's biggest rock concert to focus the attention of the world on the plight of Africa's poor.

In response to the plummeting aid levels, the United Nations introduced the Global Health Fund with the goal of raising $10 billion annually—from governments of the economically affluent countries as well as private donors—for the fight against HIV/AIDS, tuberculosis, and malaria in the developing countries. In 2002, its first year of operation, only one-tenth of the needed amount was received—once again illustrating the lack of commitment to the cause on the part of the so-called donor community. Today, as highlighted at the 2004 World AIDS Conference, the Global Health Fund continues to fall short of meeting its $10 billion annual goal. With four-fifths of the world's wealth, and only 5 percent of the world's HIV cases, the question must be asked: how can governments and individuals of the developed nations continue to ignore their moral responsibility to do all they can to significantly reduce the suffering of fellow human beings?

At the heart of all this is the old, difficult philosophical dilemma of what *are* the responsibilities of the wealthy to address the needs of the poor? Previous literature on the subject—especially on duty to aid and famine relief—provides some basic answers as to why the rich should be expected to act in the current crisis. This is especially appropriate given the fact that conditions of poverty are a major contributing factor to the level of vulnerability to HIV infection.

As S. R. Benatar and Peter A. Singer point out in their 2000 *British Medical Journal* article, "A New Look at International Research Ethics," ethical reasoning shouldn't merely follow simple prescribed rules but should consider each case as it exists in its own context, "weighing and balancing competing moral requirements and developing justifiable conclusions." So how do these classical arguments or "rules" on the relationship of the rich and the poor relate to the African AIDS crisis? Does AIDS in Africa raise any new or special issues that might compel the skeptics of such rules to believe that maybe, at least in the context of Africa and AIDS, the deaths of the poor are the responsibilities of the rich? In the light of the ever-growing problem, these discussions are critical because, if ceased or forgotten, lives will continue to be lost. However, if governments and individuals are continually reminded of the situation and their responsibility to their fellow human beings, their contributions will increase and some lives may be saved.

Singer's Ethics of Benevolence

Princeton University professor Singer is an Australian philosopher and teacher and founder of the Center for Human Bioethics at Monash University in Melbourne. His 1972 *Philosophy and Public Affairs* article, "Famine, Affluence, and Morality," is widely recognized as pioneering discussion on morality, affluence, and the needs of the poor. In writing about Singer's work in his 1994 *Ethics* article, "International Aid and the Scope of Kindness" G. Cullity says Singer has "stimulated philosophical discussion of whether affluence is immoral in a world where there is starvation." The fact that Singer's article has been reprinted more than two dozen times may just be a demonstration of its stature within philosophical circles.

In "Famine, Affluence, and Morality," Singer concludes that the affluent have an obligation to assist those whose lives are in danger, such as those living in conditions of absolute poverty. His argument is anchored in two basic principles:

Principle 1: Suffering and death from lack of food, shelter, and medical care are bad.

Principle 2: If we can prevent something bad without sacrificing anything of comparable moral significance, we ought to do it. Or, at least, if we can prevent something bad without sacrificing anything of any moral significance, we ought to do it.

The first principle—also stated simply by Singer as "absolute poverty is bad"—appears to be widely accepted. Singer says it would be hard to find any plausible ethical view that didn't regard absolute poverty as bad, especially considering its definition, which he cites in his 1979 book, *Practical Ethics*, as "a condition of life so characterized by malnutrition, illiteracy, disease, squalid surroundings, high infant mortality and low life expectancy as to be beneath any reasonable definition of human decency." John Arthur, in his 1996 article, "Rights and the Duty to Bring Aid," in W. Aiken and H. LaFollette's *World Hunger and Morality*, says Singer's first principle is "obviously true." In relation to HIV/AIDS, which is increasingly being recognized as a disease of the poor, it would seem reasonable for one to expect a broad agreement to the proposition that it is bad for African people to be dying of AIDS, almost defenseless against it because of their absolute poverty.

The question of whose responsibility it should be to offer aid in such bad situations is what the second principle attempts to answer. By the phrase *something of comparable moral significance*, Singer refers to sacrificing "without causing anything else comparably bad to happen, or doing something that is wrong in itself, or failing to promote some moral good, comparable in significance to the bad thing we can prevent." This principle, as indicated, has two versions; the latter weaker than the first. The weaker one substitutes the word *comparable* for the phrase *any moral* significance in order to reduce what Singer perceives as an incredibly high standard set by the stronger version.

Unlike the first principle, the second has attracted some controversy. Arthur, for example, has argued that such an *obligation* for the rich to give some of their wealth to those in absolute poverty contradicts their right to their private property. In talking about the rights of ownership Arthur asserts that if P acquires x, for example, in a just social arrangement without violating others' rights, then P has a special title to x that P is entitled to weigh against the desires of others. P need not, in determining whether he ought to give x to another, overlook the fact that x is his; he acquired it fairly, and so has special say in what happens to it.

In the light of this view, Arthur goes on to propose what he thinks would be the "most adequate" principle which would take into consideration the rights of the affluent: "If it is in our power to prevent death of an innocent without sacrificing anything of substantial significance then we ought morally to do it." Arthur doesn't explain exactly what determines "substantial significance" but does suggest two factors to determine whether what is given up by the affluent is of substantial significance. First, he says, the needs to be considered to be of substantial significance must be identified. These would include those things a person can't function physically without—such as food, clothing, health care, and housing. Secondly, he suggests that, "if the lack of *x* would not affect the long-term happiness of a person, then *x* is of no substantial significance" to give.

Turning this to the African HIV/AIDS crisis, it is vital to determine how much is enough to give. Here the United Nations' projected annual figure of $10 billion may reasonably be taken as the minimum beyond which the wealthy can say they have fulfilled their moral obligations to help in the AIDS crisis. Applying this figure to their differing principles may diffuse the debate between Singer and Arthur. What, and exactly how much, is of "comparable moral significance" in Singer's principle or is of "substantial significance" in Arthur's may not be relevant to HIV/AIDS when we consider how much the UN asks the affluent countries to give to the Global Health Fund. The $10 billion needed annually to produce a meaningful response to the AIDS epidemic in the developing coun-

---

Turning . . . to the African HIV/AIDS crisis, it is vital to determine how much is enough to give.

---

tries is estimated by Africa Action to constitute only 0.005 percent of the economies of the collective seven richest countries. This amount is only a minute fraction of the surplus these countries possess and is thus far too low to cause anything that could be described as "comparably bad" in the event they gave the requested amount.

With respect to the weaker version of Singer's second principle; if the 0.005 percent (or 2 cents out of $100 according to other estimates)—could be considered by anyone to be too significant to give away for such a good cause, then nothing would likely ever be considered of the right significance. Following Arthur's criteria, it is clear that meeting the needs of the poor and the HIV infected in the less affluent countries would of substantial significance. This is also consistent with conclusions drawn elsewhere that the claims of those who have urgent unmet needs simply outweigh the claims of those who possess more than they need.

The Ethics of "Letting Die"

Lifeboat ethics is a theory proposed in 1974 by bio-ethicist and ecologist Garrett Hardin that offers a general case against helping the poor. Published in *Psychology Today*, the theory divides the world into two, with two-thirds of it made up of poor nations while one-third is comprised of rich nations. The following metaphor is then used to represent the situation: the rich nations are seen collectively as a lifeboat almost full of comparatively, rich people, and the poor are represented as people swimming in the ocean, begging to be allowed into the lifeboat. The question is then asked: what should the lifeboat passengers do, given that their boat has room that could accommodate only a small proportion of those drowning outside? Hardin suggests that, to ensure their survival (and avoid drowning in case the boat's carrying capacity is exceeded or safety factors, predetermined by the manufacturers, are compromised), the rich shouldn't allow any of the swimmers into the lifeboat.

Hardin asserts in "Lifeboat Ethics: The Case Against Helping the Poor" that this is "the basic metaphor within which we must work out our solutions." But does this faithfully represent reality as we know it? According to environmental ethicist H. Rolston III, the so-called G-7 nations, which are populated by one-fifth of the world's peoples, produce and consume about four-fifths of the world's goods and services while the developing nations, with four-fifths of the world's population, produce and consume just one-fifth of the world's resources. In 1989 the richest 20 percent of the world's people received 83 percent of the global income while the poorest 20 percent only received 1.4 percent.

Lifeboat ethics becomes an excuse to continue to "let die" those who are poor, and consequently those with HIV and AIDS.

Africa, a home to more than 10 percent of global population, lives on just 1 percent of the global economy. In 1993 Richard Smith reported in "Overpopulation and Overconsumption: Combating the Two Main Drivers of Global Destruction" in the *British Medical Journal*, that people in the developing world each use 0.28 kilowatts of energy per year and those in the developed world use 3.2 kilowatts, with those in the United States using an incredible 9 kilowatts. From just these few examples one can't help but conclude—as ethicists, including J. P. Sterba in his 1996 paper "Global Justice" (in William Aiken and Hugh Lafollette's *World Hunger and Morality*), have—that "there is, still enough resources worldwide to put an end to absolute poverty. The problem is still one of distribution."

Adopting Hardin's metaphor, this conclusion tells us that the lifeboat is far from full. Lifeboat? Perhaps a more accurate metaphor would be that of an ocean liner with a handful of people on board who continue to refuse safety to near drowning people nearby. Therefore, a scenario of letting the poor die can't be applied to the issues that affect the real world and its affairs. In fact, even applied to the AIDS situation, it would be hard to see how anyone could equate the $10 billion asked for annually by the UN with begging to enter a lifeboat. The poor of the world aren't asking to live in the luxuries of the rich, nor to live with them in their own countries, but merely for the basics: food, health, and a dignified survival where they are.

In the light of such an analysis, lifeboat ethics becomes an excuse to continue to "let die" those who are poor, and consequently those with HIV and AIDS. And this is indeed what we are witnessing with the AIDS crisis. As mentioned previously, life expectancies in Africa have fallen in some countries by twenty years or more. In Botswana, for instance, the life expectancy has fallen from sixty-seven years to forty since the HIV crisis. In many sub-Saharan countries, the chances that an adolescent will ultimately die of AIDS is greater than 50 percent. Antenatal HIV prevalence has also been reported as greater than 10 percent and as much as 30 percent in some countries. What all these figures represent is the scale of premature death of Africans due to AIDS. By not supporting the UN's Global Health Fund and the other efforts that would ultimately preserve these lives, the developed countries could rightly be seen as letting the poor die. And if no moral significance exists between killing someone and letting someone die, then these deaths of the poor may indeed be viewed as a responsibility of the economically affluent.

Conclusion

In a world priding itself as civilized, the African AIDS statistics and the extent of suffering they reveal should be devastating enough to provoke those with extra resources to spontaneous benevolent action. In the absence of such compassionate spontaneity, however, resort to reason isn't an improper thing to do. I hope this article reminds us all of why the 5,000 African lives lost daily should be saved; if it isn't just because they are fellow humans then let it be because of Singer's principles of benevolence, which may rightly be seen as philosophies of hope for a dying continent. It is only a positive response to these principles by those with extra resources that will ultimately bring life to Africa, as well as communicating the warm message to the world's poor that the world is not such a cruel place after all.

The Church & AIDS in Africa

Condoms & the Culture of Life

By Marcella Alsan
Commonweal April 21, 2006

As a young physician, I often second-guess myself. In practicing medicine such self-criticism is warranted, even obligatory, because a wrong diagnosis can lead to misguided therapy and may end in death. After working at a Catholic hospital in the small sub-Saharan country of Swaziland, however, there is one diagnosis I pronounce with uncharacteristic certitude: AIDS.

The typical patient is a young woman between eighteen and thirty years of age. She is wheeled into the examining room in a hospital chair or dragged in, supported by her sister, aunt, or brother. She is frequently delirious; her face is gaunt; her limbs look like desiccated twigs. Surprisingly, the young woman is already a mother many times over, yet she will not live to see her children grow up. More shocking still, she is married; her husband infected her with the deadly virus.

This is the reality: a married woman living in Southern Africa is at higher risk of becoming infected with HIV than an unmarried woman. Extolling abstinence and fidelity, as the Catholic Church does, will not protect her; in all likelihood she is already monogamous. It is her husband who is likely to have HIV. Yet refusing a husband's sexual overtures risks ostracism, violence, and destitution for herself and her children. Given these realities, isn't opposing the use of condoms tantamount to condemning countless women to death? In the midst of the AIDS epidemic, which has already killed tens of millions and preys disproportionately on the poor, the condom acts as a *contra mortem* and its use is justified by the Catholic consistent ethic of life.

At least, this is the view of many Catholics at the front lines of the global HIV battle. Catholic organizations mercifully provide around 25 percent of the care AIDS victims receive worldwide. Many of the clergy and laity involved in treating people with AIDS, who otherwise fully ascribe to the church's teachings on sexual ethics and the sanctity of marriage, nevertheless endorse the use of condoms. They argue that the preservation of human life is paramount. Fr. Valeriano Paitoni, working in São Paulo, Brazil, summarized this perspective: "AIDS is a world epidemic, a public-health problem that must be confronted with scientific advances and methods that have proven effective," he says. "Rejecting condom use is to oppose the fight for life."

Bishop Kevin Dowling of South Africa has also been imploring the Vatican to view condom use as curtailing the transmission of death rather than precluding the transmission of life. In South Africa, 5.3 million people are infected with HIV and 25 percent of all pregnant women test positive for the virus. Dowling prays that the Holy Spirit will intervene to change minds in Rome. He believes Pope Benedict XVI's view on the use of condoms would change, "if his visits to poor countries were done in such a way that he could sit in a shack and see a young mother dying of AIDS with her baby." Not long ago, Belgian Cardinal Godfried Danneels stated on Dutch television that although sex with a person infected with HIV is to be avoided, "if it should take place, the person must use a condom in order not to disobey the commandment condemning murder, in addition to breaking the commandment which forbids adultery." He added: "Protecting oneself against sickness or death is an act of prevention. Morally, it cannot be judged on the same level as when a condom is used to reduce the number of births."

Unfortunately, the Vatican has not budged. Condoms thwart conception; therefore, by the 1968 encyclical *Humanae vitae*, their use is proscribed. End of debate. In a 2003 Vatican document titled *Family Values Versus Safe Sex*, the use of condoms in HIV-prevention programs was forcefully rejected:

> The Catholic bishops of South Africa, Botswana, and Swaziland categorically regard the widespread and indiscriminate promotion of condoms as an immoral and misguided weapon in our battle against HIV/AIDS for the following reasons. The use of condoms goes against human dignity. Condoms change the beautiful act of love into a selfish search for pleasure—while rejecting responsibility. Condoms do not guarantee protection against HIV/AIDS. Condoms may even be one of the main reasons for the spread of HIV/AIDS.

Cardinal Alfonso Lopez Trujillo, head of the Pontifical Council for the Family, has elaborated on the latter point: "In the case of the AIDS virus, which is around 450 times smaller than the sperm cell, the condom's latex material obviously gives much less security . . . to talk of condoms as 'safe sex' is a form of Russian roulette." Trujillo called on ministries of health to require "a warning, that the condom is not safe" on packages distributed worldwide.

Although it is true that condoms are not 100-percent effective in preventing HIV infection, they do reduce the risk of transmission significantly. Comparing condom use to a suicidal dare, as Cardinal Trujillo does, is scientifically inaccurate and socially irresponsible. A preponderance of medical research demonstrates that condoms help prevent the spread of HIV. For example, the European Study Group on Heterosexual Transmission of HIV followed 124 discordant couples (in which only one of the pair is infected with HIV) who consistently used condoms. Over a two-year period and roughly fifteen thousand sexual acts, none of the HIV-negative partners contracted the virus. Thai investigators examining the impact of condom use among the military reported that new infections dropped from 12.5 percent in 1993 to 6.7 percent in 1995. The number of new HIV infections in Thailand plummeted after the introduction of a "100-percent condom use" program. Uganda earned its reputation as a paragon of HIV prevention for its now-famous ABC program: Abstain, Be faithful, and Consistent, Correct use of Condoms. Following the implementation of ABC, HIV infection in Uganda decreased from between 15 and 20 percent of the population in the early 1990s to 5 percent in 2003. A comparative analysis of Ugandan population-based surveys in 1989 and 1995 concluded that delaying the age of first sexual encounters, decreasing the number of casual partners, *and* increasing condom use all contributed to Uganda's success. More recently, though, HIV has been on the rise in Uganda. Current data estimate 7 percent of the popula-

---

The Vatican must be made aware that abstaining from sex is not a choice that many women living in the developing world have.

---

tion is infected with the AIDS virus. Some advocacy groups attribute this upswing to a national condom shortage orchestrated by the Ugandan government under pressure from the Bush administration. The Health Ministry of Uganda refutes this allegation, stating that delays in the distribution of condoms have been the result of enhanced inspection of shipments after a batch of Chinese condoms was purportedly discovered to be faulty.

Of course, never having sex will significantly reduce the risk of contracting a sexually transmitted disease. (It will not, though, completely eliminate the risk of contracting HIV, since the virus is also transmitted via blood products, birthing, and breastfeeding.) But the Vatican must be made aware that abstaining from sex is *not* a choice that many women living in the developing world have. To preach fidelity and abstinence assumes that a woman can determine with whom she sleeps and when—a grave misunderstanding of the relations between the sexes in places where women are sometimes betrothed at birth or sold for cattle. How can the Vatican continue to prohibit the use of a life-saving intervention amid a pandemic of unprecedented proportions? By reflexively invoking *Humane vitae* whenever the condom issue arises, the church has tragically misdiagnosed the moral problem at hand.

Benedict XVI made his first comments as pope regarding condom use at a June 2005 papal audience. His listeners included bishops from South Africa, Swaziland, Botswana, Namibia, and Lesotho.

After reviewing the importance of catechesis and recruiting African men to the priesthood, the pope turned his attention to AIDS: "It is of great concern that the fabric of African life, its very source of hope and stability, is threatened by divorce, abortion, prostitution, human trafficking, and a contraception mentality." He emphasized that contraception leads to a "breakdown in sexual morality." In the speech, the pope made a diagnosis: condoms increase sexual immorality, and sexual immorality increases the spread of AIDS. The logical treatment for sexual immorality is Christian marriage, fidelity, and chastity. Cardinal Javier Lozano Barragan, president of the Vatican's Council for Pastoral Assistance to Health Care Workers, had reached a similar conclusion in his Message for World AIDS Day (December 1, 2003): "We have to present this [lifestyles emphasizing marriage, fidelity, and chastity] as the main way for the effective prevention of infection and spread of HIV/AIDS, since the phenomenon of AIDS is a pathology of the spirit."

> Young brides are acquiring HIV from their husbands, who tend to be many years older and were infected before marriage.

Fidelity in marriage and abstinence for everyone else would be the only indicated intervention if a "pathological spirit" were the only cause of AIDS. Unfortunately, many victims of HIV are blameless. Currently, 25 million HIV-infected individuals and 12 million AIDS orphans are living in sub-Saharan Africa. The communities hardest hit by AIDS are among the world's most impoverished. Sub-Saharan Africa, which has the world's lowest per capita annual income ($450 US), and where half of all individuals live in extreme poverty (earning less than a dollar a day), is ground zero of the epidemic. Over 70 percent of all infections, 80 percent of all AIDS-related deaths, and 90 percent of all AIDS-orphanings occur here. And with over six thousand new infections per day, the epidemic shows no signs of abating.

Obviously, the poor are limited in their access to education and to health services. Ignorance kills. When accurate information is not available, myths multiply. Surveys from forty countries indicate that more than 50 percent of young people aged fifteen to twenty-four have serious misconceptions about how HIV/AIDS is transmitted. Research by the Nelson Mandela Foundation has shown that 35 percent of twelve- to fourteen-year-olds thought that sex with a virgin could cure AIDS, or were unsure whether or not that statement was true. In other impoverished nations, AIDS is thought to be spread by witchcraft, mosquito bites, or through polio vaccination.

As already noted, the church in Africa is facing a grim reality even when it comes to sex in marriage. According to UNICEF, teenage brides in some African countries are becoming infected with the AIDS virus at higher rates than sexually active unmarried girls of similar ages. That's because young brides are acquiring HIV from their husbands, who tend to be many years older and were infected before marriage. Clearly, abstinence and fidelity prevention strategies will not reliably protect these women. The result is reflected in the epidemiology of the disease: more than two-thirds of new HIV infections among people aged fifteen to twenty-five occur among women. In some areas of Africa, girls are five to six times more likely to be HIV-positive than boys of the same age.

The suffering associated with these alarming trends is difficult to comprehend. Stephen Lewis, UN special envoy for HIV/AIDS in Africa, summarized it this way: "To this catalogue of horrors, there must be added, in the case of Africa, that the pandemic is now, conclusively and irreversibly, a ferocious assault on women and girls." What has been called the "feminization of poverty" is a particularly lethal phenomenon in conjunction with AIDS. Gender discrimination in much of the world prohibits women from owning property or earning a living wage. To survive these harsh economic realities, many women are forced into prostitution. Paul Farmer, the Harvard physician and anthropologist, has noted that the women he interviewed in Haiti "were straightforward about the nonvoluntary aspect of their sexual activity: in their opinions, poverty had forced them into unfavorable unions. Under such conditions, one wonders what to make of the notion of 'consensual sex.'"

In Africa, the legacy of colonial racism, and especially of apartheid, still plays a role in determining one's risk of contracting HIV. In South Africa, a migrant labor system separated husbands from wives and made normal family life impossible. That pattern continues in the mining industry today, where the conflation of harsh working conditions, separation from wife and family, and the invariable proximity of brothels facilitate the spread of HIV from sex worker to laborer, and thence to his wife and children.

Acknowledging the role that poverty, racism, and gender inequality play in fueling the spread of AIDS in no way diminishes the need for personal responsibility and moral restraint. Indeed, even the correct and consistent use of condoms will require behavior change and individual accountability. But by narrowly diagnosing AIDS as a problem of morality and by discrediting a vital component of HIV prevention, the church is advancing a remedy that is woefully inadequate. In medicine, partial therapy is at best ineffective—and at worst lethal.

If men did not stray, if women had rights, if AIDS did not kill, perhaps the church's strict ban on condom use would be morally defensible. But none of these conditions applies in Africa today. As a consequence, the cost of the church's inflexibility may mean not only untold human suffering, but the loss of millions of innocent lives.

To Tackle a Taboo

How Africa Is Opening Up a New Front in the Fight Against AIDS

BY ANDREW JACK
FINANCIAL TIMES, JANUARY 18, 2007

It was no surprise to Sibongile when her husband died of Aids in 2003, even though he had always refused to take a test. She had suspected that he was HIV positive ever since she learnt of the death of one of his girlfriends two years earlier.

"I was expecting it. He was a real ladies' man," she says with an embarrassed smile. "I knew it for a long time but I stayed. I really loved him and he helped me financially. One of the things in our culture is that you don't question your husband."

Her experience in Swaziland touches on a taboo that a growing number of public health experts believe must be breached if the devastating impact of HIV is to be reversed in southern Africa: the need to change sexual behaviour and, above all, to reduce the number of sexual partners people have.

While the emphasis in the fight against Aids in the developing world since the turn of the millennium has focused on increasing the number of people on treatment, such efforts do nothing to stem the continued rise in new infections.

Although hundreds of millions of dollars of donor and local funding have poured into HIV prevention programmes, far less effort has gone into persuading people to change their sexual practices. "Prevention has concentrated on testing, condoms, safe blood and mother-to-child transmission—things that fall easily off bureaucrats' lips," says Derek von Wissell, who runs Nercha, Swaziland's official National Emergency Response Council on HIV/Aids. "Behaviour change is the difficult side. It needs a whole societal shift."

Recent initiatives in his country and others in the region reflect a new determination to tackle a sensitive subject. The debate has long been politicised. Thabo Mbeki, president of South Africa, was among those who argued that advocates who linked Aids to promiscuity were propagating racist sexual stereotypes of Africans.

In the US and elsewhere, the debate around prevention became polarised around which aspects of the mantra of "ABC"—"abstinence, be faithful and condomise"—should receive priority. Religious groups focused on the first two in an effort to promote more conservative sexuality. More socially liberal advocates argued above all for condoms, maintaining that it was unrealistic to expect A and B to work.

Pepfar, US President George W. Bush's programme of Aids assistance to the developing world, was caught in the middle. Inspired by his alliance with the religious right, its mandate required substantial funds to go to promoting abstinence and fidelity—even though it is also spending considerable amounts on condoms, too.

"When you say ABC, it immediately conjures up George Bush," says Daniel Halperin from Harvard's School of Public Health, who specialises in Aids and behaviour change. "There was an immediate polarisation between those saying condoms were evil and those who argued that only condoms were good."

He helped co-ordinate a letter two years ago to The Lancet, the medical journal, stressing the need for an evidence-based approach. It was signed by leading figures including President Yoweri Museveni of Uganda and Archbishop Desmond Tutu of South Africa. But opinion is changing only gradually—and funding more slowly still.

Mr Halperin and other public health specialists argue that, while all three approaches to prevention have a role in the fight against Aids, changing sexual behaviour and reducing the number of partners has been the "neglected middle child" in ABC.

In countries such as Thailand, Cambodia and Brazil, emphasis on the use of condoms was central to tackling infection rates. But Mark Dybul, the head of Pepfar, argues that the decline was also driven by a fall in the number of men visiting prostitutes—the key driver of the epidemic in those regions.

In southern Africa, Aids has a different pattern. It is not concentrated, as elsewhere, in a few high-risk groups such as sex workers and their clients, intravenous drug users or gay men. It is instead a generalised epidemic, helping explain why the region accounts for two-fifths both of all Aids cases and of new infections.

"Applying lessons (of condom use) from a concentrated epidemic to a region where there is a generalised epidemic was bordering on scientific insanity," says Mr Dybul. "We have not listened enough to Africans. It is tough to find one who doesn't say A, B and C is what we need."

There is no single or satisfactory explanation for why HIV in southern Africa—which has infected up to 40 per cent of the adult population in Swaziland and nearby Lesotho—is so much higher than in the rest of the world. Poverty, malnutrition, lack of circumcision and the low status of women play a strong part. However, a growing body of evidence points to the predominant role of one aspect of sexual behaviour.

As far as research into such sensitive questions can be relied on, many aspects of African sexuality mirror practices elsewhere. The average total number of sexual partners a person has in a lifetime may even be lower than in many western countries. But in much of the region, men and women often have several concurrent sexual partners over months or years.

In countries such as Swaziland, which traditionally practised polygamy and where King Mswati himself has 13 wives, it is almost institutionalised. Elsewhere in the region it is widespread—though rarely discussed in public.

The practice sharply intensifies the spread of the epidemic for at least two reasons. First, HIV's ability to be transmitted reaches a peak in the weeks after someone has been infected. So those in multiple partnerships can rapidly spread the disease to others.

With one study in Malawi suggesting that in seven villages, 65 per cent of sexually active adults were linked into a single network, such concurrence means HIV can quickly spread across entire communities.

> There is no single or satisfactory explanation for why HIV in southern Africa . . . is so much higher than in the rest of the world.

A second explanation is that long-term sexual partners, who show greater trust in and commitment to each other, are far less likely to use condoms. That also increases the likelihood that if one is HIV positive, the infection will be eventually passed on to the other.

The importance of such patterns of behaviour are beginning to be recognised. Public health specialists convened last year by the Southern African Development Community concluded in a report: "Key drivers of the epidemic in southern Africa . . . included multiple concurrent partnerships by men and women with low consistent condom use." It highlighted instances where HIV infections appeared to be falling and linked these to successful programmes aimed at changing behaviour, notably in Kenya, Uganda and Zimbabwe.

Why has it taken public health professionals so long to reach this conclusion? One reason is the complexity of establishing the link. Drug trials can often quickly and clearly demonstrate a quantifiable effect of taking a medicine. Behavioural studies are much more complex. Efforts to change sexual behaviour may take many years to have any effect—and the impact on reduced HIV can often be attributed to a range of factors other than prevention programmes.

Perhaps most importantly, few programmes specifically intended to change behaviour have taken place—and fewer still have focused directly on reducing the number of partners. That reflects ideology, the sensitivity of the subject and a distaste for the social coercion attempted in programmes such as Uganda's "zero grazing" initiative in the late 1980s, in which local councils assumed powers to monitor young people's sexual activity.

The lack of behaviour-change programmes also mirrors a concentration by funders and doctors on medicines and other "technological" solutions to Aids. Purnima Mane, director of policy evidence and partnerships at UNAids, the United Nations' Aids agency, says:

"In the last 10 years, the focus has been highly biomedical. Social scientists have withdrawn a bit. They have been seen as playing second fiddle."

Furthermore, when programmes have been launched, monitoring and evaluation has often been lacking. "We have launched boutique projects rather than scaling things up," she says. "We don't establish what makes them effective. That has been the tragedy, because we have wanted to act quickly."

Warren Parker, a public health consultant based in Johannesburg, is more blunt. "It's very frustrating that so much money is going to imbeciles," he says. "Everyone is putting money into youth programmes but we've been much less focused on partner reduction."

He was an outspoken critic of loveLife, a glitzy South African programme targeted at young people, which received tens of millions of dollars in support from agencies including the Kaiser Foundation in the US and the Global Fund to fight Aids, TB and Malaria. Disappointment with the ineffective and poorly managed scheme eventually led the Fund to cut short its support.

With so little data available, making the case for partner-reduction programmes is only the beginning. Ms Purnima argues: "People have often shied away even from presenting the message because of the sensitivities of language and culture."

Roger Kunene, who is studying for the priesthood, who works with Aids orphans in Swaziland, highlights the absence of role models. "In our culture, you have to have a lot of girlfriends to be a man," he says. "Many people don't practise what they preach. A lot of teachers warn about Aids but are having relationships with their pupils."

Swaziland has been one of the boldest recent experimenters, launching a media campaign last year denouncing the widespread practice of having "secret lovers." It quickly ran into controversy, accused by local HIV activists of stigmatising sufferers, and toned down its approach within two weeks.

But polls afterwards suggested that most people across the country knew about the campaign, the majority supported it and a significant proportion claimed that it would influence them to reduce their number of partners.

Behavioural change programmes will provide only a partial solution to tackling Aids in southern Africa and other heavily affected parts of the world. As has been seen in the developed world, "disinhibition" can set in, causing infection rates to rise again. "The messages get old, people get sick of them and are not afraid of dying any more," says Mr Dybul.

> Behavioural change programmes will provide only a partial solution to tackling Aids in southern Africa and other heavily affected parts of the world.

But there is a growing sense that partner reduction should receive far greater support and evaluation than it has so far, supplementing a growing number of medical and other approaches. These include increased HIV testing, counselling and malecircumcision.

"We need to create a rising tide of societal change," says Nercha's Mr von Wissell. "My gut feeling is that behaviour change works. While all these academics are talking, we have to act."

Giving Away HIV Drugs Is Not as Easy as It Seems

AIDS Alert, November 1, 2001

When officials with a German pharmaceutical firm announced in July 2000 that the company would make its HIV antiretroviral drug nevirapine (Viramune) available to any pregnant women in sub-Saharan Africa who need it for the prevention of mother-to-child transmission (MTCT) of HIV, they thought their biggest problem would be to meet the flood of demand.

They were wrong.

"When we began, we thought our supply chain would be overwhelmed by the number of requests," says John Wecker, PhD, an HIV specialist and coordinator of HIV activities in the developing world for Boehringer Ingelheim of Ingelheim, Germany.

"What happened was that in the end it turned out we've given away very little drug to date, although it is increasing," Wecker says. "The major obstacle has been the lack of quality health care capacity within most of these developing countries."

Boehringer Ingelheim's experiences can serve as both a model for and a lesson to other drug manufacturers who plan to make HIV medications available at no or very low cost to the developing nations hit hardest by the pandemic.

"Preventing mother-to-child transmission is not just having the drugs available; it's much more," says Dirk Buyse, MD, international program officer for the Elizabeth Glaser Pediatric AIDS Foundation in Washington, DC.

"The essential components are, first, to have voluntary testing and counseling on HIV and MTCT," Buyse says. "When you look at an MTCT program, the cost of the drug component is less than 5% of the total budget of the MTCT program."

Programs that seek to prevent MTCT also could serve as models and leaders for future HIV antiretroviral therapy treatment in the developing world, says Connie Osborne, MB.Ch.B, the MTCT voluntary counseling and testing focal point for UNAIDS in Geneva, Switzerland.

"Initially, we were overly enthusiastic and we thought countries would just jump at it, but MTCT programs in developing countries are relatively new," Osborne says.

Now as more pregnant women are being reached through the programs that will distribute free nevirapine, perhaps the next step will be to provide follow-up care to these women so they might also receive antiretroviral therapy, Osborne says.

UNAIDS is promoting such an extension of MTCT prevention programs through its new MTC Plus initiative, which advocates drugs for the treatment of mothers who are living with HIV. This may also help slow the sub-Saharan region's tremendous growth in orphans.

But none of these programs are cheap or easy, as Boehringer Ingelheim has learned.

In the case of providing nevirapine, an economic analysis by Boehringer Ingelheim and the German government showed that to prevent MTCT in Uganda, Kenya, and Tanzania, the value of the drug represented only 1.2% of the total investment needed to establish MTCT programs, Wecker says.

The other expenses come from identifying, hiring, and training counselors; making physical/medical services available; providing necessary transportation and information to bring pregnant women into the health care system; providing women with antenatal care; providing nevirapine therapy; and providing quality postnatal care, Wecker says.

Then there's the issue of infant feeding: Is it safer for women to nurse their babies, even when there's the potential for transmitting HIV, or do women have clean water available with which to mix infant formula?

However, as Boehringer Ingelheim officials learned, the key is to take what little infrastructure is available and work with it.

The German pharmaceutical company has begun to work with nongovernmental organizations (NGOs), physicians, charitable organizations, and others who directly provide health care services to the poor in developing nations. Also, the company hired Axios International of Dublin, Ireland, to organize the distribution of nevirapine to sub-Saharan Africa.

"When we went to the NGO level, we heard that the number of applications for the drug will begin to increase dramatically," Wecker says. "And so that's one thing Axios will do for us: Help us manage the sheer load of applications we're hoping to get."

Axios will ensure that the requests for nevirapine match the organization's ability to distribute the drug, says Joseph Saba, MD, chief executive officer of Axios.

"We basically open the dialogue in programs, discuss ethical issues, and make sure we're comfortable that these programs have established an infrastructure and will be able to implement what they say they can implement," Saba explains.

"Many of these programs have a good idea and are well thought through," Saba adds. "But some of them are coming from people who have their hearts in the right place and want to do something, but they don't have experience in calculating doses correctly."

There have been examples of programs in a country where the HIV prevalence rate is 6% that made a forecast of needing 20,000 doses of nevirapine. Then when the situation was further explored, it was discovered that the program really could only handle 800 doses at the start, Saba says.

"We don't want drugs expiring on the shelves," Saba adds.

The logistics of distributing even a simple therapy of nevirapine can be difficult. The therapy to prevent MTCT of HIV involves giving the pregnant woman one 200 mg tablet during labor, followed by a less than one milliliter of suspension drug given to the infant within 72 hours after birth, Wecker says.

But here is where such simple therapy for an affluent nation becomes complicated for a poor country: The pregnant woman may see a physician at some point before her due date, but there is little guarantee that the woman will return to the same clinic when she is in labor, Saba says.

Further complications involve the fact that only an estimated 5% to 10% of pregnant women in sub-Saharan Africa and other parts of the developing world know whether they are HIV-positive, and their clinicians have no fast way to discover their serostatus as the women go into labor. This means that for a drug giveaway program to prevent MTCT successfully, it would need to include testing and counseling facilities for pregnant women.

"They would need to hire counselors and very simply have a private room where the counselor can sit down with the women and discuss HIV and testing, and then, with HIV-positive women, explain to them what it means to be HIV-positive and how they can get help," Saba says.

Now, more than a year since beginning the program, Boehringer Ingelheim is making progress in distributing the drug to pregnant women. So far there are 19 projects in 12 countries that are part of the Viramune Donation Program for the prevention of MTCT, and these projects have ordered enough drug to treat 49,800 mother-child pairs. The countries involved include Congo Brazzaville, Ghana, Guyana, Kenya, Namibia, Nigeria, Rwanda, Senegal, Sierra Leone, Uganda, Zambia, and Zimbabwe.

Wecker's advice to other pharmaceutical companies offering free or deeply discounted antiretroviral drugs to poor nations is to anticipate these types of infrastructure problems before starting the program.

"You can't underestimate the lack of health care capacity," Wecker says. "Whenever you set your goals, you have to take into consideration the realism and the reality of what's there and what's not there."

II. HIV/AIDS AND ITS EFFECTS ON WOMEN AND ORPHANED CHILDREN

Editor's Introduction

According to UNAIDS three quarters of HIV-positive Africans between the ages of 15 and 24 are women. A variety of factors contribute to this phenomenon. Often, out of economic necessity, men travel far from their homes to find work. Given this excess of migrant male labor, sex workers are common. Condom use, however, remains taboo in many areas. Thus HIV/AIDS can spread rapidly. After being exposed to the virus, the men subsequently return home and put their families at risk. Due to the predominantly patriarchal family structure, wives have little with which to protect themselves. Indeed, demanding their husbands use condoms or refusing sex altogether can lead to violence.

In the first article in this chapter, "Violence Against Women Complicated HIV/AIDS Struggle," a reporter for the Inter Press Service argues that unless women gain more power in determining their sexual relationships, the spread of HIV will continue. Though certain countries have passed statutes to deter violence against women, laws alone are not enough, the writer contends. Rather education must be employed to persuade men to join the struggle for gender equality.

An estimated 250,000 women were raped during the Rwandan genocide of 1994. As a result, many of them became infected with HIV/AIDS. A writer for *Africa Renewal*, in "Rwandan Women: AIDS Therapy Beyond Drugs," cites the examples of these women in outlining a new strategy to fight the disease. Noting that many of these victims could not participate in ARV therapy because they couldn't afford the food that had to be taken with the drugs, the author contends that hunger and poverty must be addressed throughout Africa in order to make this form of treatment more feasible.

Among the heartbreaking side effects of the AIDS epidemic in Africa are the countless orphaned children, who have not only watched their parents waste away from the disease, but are now left to face the world on their own. In this chapter's third article, "A Tale of Two Worlds," Peter Gyves notes the disproportionate number of HIV-infected women relative to men, especially in sub-Saharan Africa, but he focuses principally on the children left behind. He observes that some AIDS orphans are infected with the virus themselves, and that in the past these children were viewed as "lost causes." They often went untreated as many believed that the limited supply of ARVs should be saved for adults.

In "AIDS Orphans," Oksana Kim discusses the recently released World Health Report that focused on this troubling world phenomenon. The problem is especially acute in sub-Saharan Africa, where, according to the UN, over 2 million children are HIV positive and millions more are living without parents.

Violence Against Women
Complicated HIV/Aids Struggle

BY JOYCE MULAMA
INTER PRESS SERVICE, JANUARY 24, 2007

The issue of violence exacerbating the spread of HIV/Aids, particularly in women, has remained a hot one at the World Social Forum (WSF), taking place here this week.

From Africa to Asia, activists are reiterating that violence against women remains a threat to the HIV/Aids fight, and that without governments addressing the matter, winning the war against the disease will be an uphill task.

"Violence is largely a cause of HIV infection among many women; violence in the homes and in the streets, violence everywhere," says Ludfine Anyango, the national HIV/Aids coordinator at Action Kenya-International.

The fact that women do not have an upper hand in negotiating their sexual relationships exposes them to the risk of being infected with the disease, agreed Forum participants.

"Many women cannot even choose when to have sex or not. Many cannot ask their husbands to use a condom because in addition to being thought as unfaithful, they fear being beaten. The woman then has no choice but to continue having unprotected sex with her spouse," Anyango added.

Violence in the streets similarly subjects female sex workers to the risk of HIV infection, according to Ros Sokunthy of Women's Agenda for Change, an organisation fighting for the rights of women, including female sex workers, in Cambodia.

"A sex worker negotiates with one man. When she gets to the venue she finds more than one man and they all want to have sex with her. When she refuses, she is beaten or raped," Sokunthy told IPS.

"Usually the sex worker has two condoms. If at the venue she finds three or four men, the condoms will not be enough. The men will beat her up if she denies them sex, or insist on using sugar plastic bags which are weak and easily get torn, exposing her to HIV infection," she said.

These scenarios, according to experts, explain why more women than men are infected with HIV/Aids. Last year's report of the United Nations Joint Programme on HIV/Aids (UNAids) says in sub-Saharan Africa—which is home to about 64 percent of the world population living with HIV/Aids—more women are infected than men.

WSF participants also heard that women were beaten by their spouses if it was discovered that they had visited HIV/Aids voluntary testing and counselling centres (VCTs).

> *Male involvement in the fight against the pandemic is critical, say groups including UNAIDS*

"We have had cases whereby some women come to us and tell us 'please do not tell my husband that I was here because if he knows, he will kill me when I go back home.' When we follow up, we find out that the husband is HIV positive," said Mary Watiti, a counsellor at a VCT centre in Kibera, Kenya's biggest slum.

"This fear discourages many women from knowing their HIV status and thus continue having unprotected sex with their spouses," she added.

This phenomenon has resuscitated calls for new laws to address all forms of violence against women, and strict implementation of the law in countries where such legislation is already on the book. Changing laws is soon as one of the effective ways of countering the spread of HIV/Aids.

Kenya came into the spotlight for having a law that addressed sexual violence, but which had loopholes that made it possible for women to continue being violated sexually, with little recourse for justice.

"Even though we have the Sexual Offences Act, it does not recognise marital rape; yet HIV/Aids is mostly spread through relationships," said Inviolata Mbwavi, the national coordinator of the Network of People Living with HIV/Aids in Kenya.

A domestic violence bill, which stipulated strict penalties for offenders in the East African country, was overtaken by time and has now to be re-tabled in parliament. The bill was introduced in 2000.

However, laws alone are not enough to address HIV/AIDS. Male involvement in the fight against the pandemic is critical, say groups including UNAIDS, given that men are generally not proactive in terms of seeking VCT services and, sometimes, compromise the management and care of those infected.

HIV/Aids experts argue that because men seem to fear stigma more than women do, they rarely visit VCT centres.

A study conducted in Indonesia last month shows that nine out of 10 men were offended when asked by their partner to go for VCT and refused testing, while eight out of 10 women agreed to be tested.

"This is because men keep thinking that VCT and HIV/AIDS is only for the high-risk groups," Suksma Ratri of Rumah Cemara, an HIV/Aids research organisation, told IPS.

Failure to seek counselling and testing locks men out from treatment programmes. This may lead to infected men taking some of medicine from their wives who are on treatment programmes.

This practice is widespread in low income settings across African countries, according to James Kamau, coordinator of the Africa Civil Society Coalition on HIV/Aids.

"Experiences in Kibera slum and the poorest areas in central and western Kenya indicate that women were sharing drugs," he said.

But experts warn that tampering with ARV (antiretrovirals, the main treatment for HIV/Aids) dosage is a sure way developing resistance to cheaper and affordable drugs. When this happens, the affected person will be forced to pay ten times more to buy ARVs that can manage resistant strains of the virus.

"As long as our men are not part of the war, then we should forget about ending HIV/Aids infection and the violence that comes with it," according to Lilian Musang'u, a WSF participant from Malawi.

The WSF is an annual gathering of social activists seeking to chart out ways of countering the dominance of the rich western nations. This meet of tens of thousands of activists generally takes place in January, as a counterweight to the World Economic Forum, an annual meeting of powerful business and political elites held in the Swiss alpine resort of Davos.

Since 2001, the events have been held in Brazil and India. Last year it was a polycentric forum that was held in three places, Bamako, Mali; Caracas, Venezuela; and Karachi, Pakistan. At least 50,000 from across the world people are present at the Nairobi event.

Rwandan Women: AIDS Therapy Beyond Drugs

By Stephanie Urdang
Africa Renewal, June 1, 2006

For Grace and her daughter Juliette, the anniversary of the April 1994 Rwanda genocide means one thing: they have lived with HIV for a dozen years, and their disease has progressed to AIDS. Grace was among the estimated 250,000 women who were raped at the time and is one of the untold numbers of women who were infected with HIV as a result. Juliette, now eight years old, is also infected.

Until recently Grace was living in abject poverty, trying to cope with the stigma associated with being HIV-positive and with the daily worry that there would be no one to look after Juliette after her early death.

At first, when Grace began to get sick, she found it inconceivable that she had AIDS. Those who carried out the genocide "murdered my husband and left me to die slowly from their AIDS," she said. She found it equally inconceivable that there were drugs that could fight the disease. "In my case, only God, who knows that it wasn't my fault that I caught this sickness, could perform a miracle and heal me."

Grace and her daughter, like Josiane, Didacienne, Triphonie and other women in her situation, have now found that they do not have to wait for miracles to occur. All have been able to benefit from the Rwandan government's commitment to providing anti-retroviral (ARV) therapy to those who need it—and for those who cannot afford it, at no cost.

These women are among the estimated 6 million Africans living with HIV/AIDS who are in immediate need of anti-retroviral medicines, out of a total of nearly 26 million HIV-positive people in the region.

Recent data from Rwanda's 2005 Demographic Health Survey indicates an estimated overall adult infection rate of 3 per cent nationally. Earlier estimates by the Joint UN Programme on HIV/AIDS (UNAIDS) for 2003 placed the prevalence rate in the towns at 6.4 per cent and in the rural areas at 2.8 per cent. The programme's *Global Report* for 2004, also using 2003 figures, estimated that some 250,000 Rwandan children and adults up to the age of 49 are living with HIV (figures for adults over 49 were not available). Of those, 22,000 were estimated to be children under the age of 15. Of particular concern is the high prevalence rate among young women between the ages of 15 and 24, five times the rate among young men of the same age group.

Wide Treatment Coverage

The Rwandan government, with financial support from a variety of sources including the Global Fund for AIDS, Tuberculosis and Malaria, the World Health Organization, the World Bank, bilateral donor agencies and private funds such as the Clinton Foundation, is able to provide ARV treatment to about 40 per cent of the people in need. Doctors and nurses are being trained, and a growing number of health clinics are able to treat AIDS patients. The estimated 19,000 people living with AIDS under treatment by December 2005 represented one of the highest coverage rates in sub-Saharan Africa.

This is particularly impressive in a country where 66 per cent of the population live below the poverty line and where the majority of households are unable to produce enough to feed themselves, even though 91 per cent rely on agriculture for their livelihoods. Rwanda's food crisis remains chronic. It is even more severe in the context of HIV/AIDS, presenting a challenge to the ultimate success of the government's treatment and care programme.

That programme involves not only medical and resource questions, but also interlocking issues of poverty, stigma and gender inequality. Because of these issues, access to ARVs is often not a reality for those who are the most marginalized and in greatest need of the medicines.

Poverty means going hungry. Hunger leads to malnutrition and a more rapid breakdown of the immune system. Social stigma against those with the disease means that many do not get tested in the first place. And gender inequality puts burdens on women that they cannot shake off on their own. Those burdens include responsibility for caring for children and other family members, ensuring that limited food supplies go first to hungry children and the risk of abandonment by men when an HIV-positive status is disclosed. Pivotal to all these issues is the need for food, a need as urgent as the drugs themselves.

Food a Daily Challenge

Sister Speciosa, a nurse and nun, is confronted with the reality of food every day as she provides treatment, care and counselling to AIDS patients at Butare Hospital, two hours drive from Kigali. "It is not only that they need the food to take with the medicine and that they need to eat more than they did when they were sick to get healthy," she says. "It's that their appetite increases. Some of my patients say they don't want to take the medicine because it makes them so hungry."

Although eligible for free tests and medication because of their lack of income, many find that the daily circumstances of their lives make it impossible for them to use those services. The lack of food or money for transport, difficult housing conditions, pervasive stigma, the stress of believing they will die without providing for their children's care—all serve to accelerate a downward spiral into despair and hinder their access to ARV drugs, even when those drugs are free. Because women are primarily responsible for feeding their children and their families, they are most deeply affected by this inability.

Dr. Anita Asiimwe, coordinator for care and treatment at the Treatment and Research AIDS Centre, a government agency, also cited the food question in an interview with *Africa Renewal*. "It is clinically established that patients need to take their drugs with food," she said. "It's a dilemma for us, as *everyone needs* food. Is it right to only provide food for those on the drugs? What about everyone else who doesn't have enough to eat?"

She illustrated her point with an anecdote about a child whose mother couldn't afford to send her to school. The child, knowing that children of people living with AIDS had their school expenses covered, asked her mother why she wasn't HIV-infected so that she could go to school too.

"Would women," Dr. Asiimwe wondered aloud, "be encouraged to become infected in order to feed their children?" At times, she says, she has to try not to be despondent about the difficulty of providing for all those in need. "I have to remind myself," she said, "of how far we have come, and not despair about how far we still have to go."

> Social stigma against those with the disease means that many do not get tested in the first place.

"We Cannot Eat Pictures"

The Ministry of Health's Nutrition Unit is fully aware of the need for a healthy diet for people living with AIDS, whether they are being treated with ARVs or not. In a recent interview for an assessment financed by the UN Development Fund for Women (UNIFEM) and undertaken by African Rights, a non-governmental organization, the ministry's secretary-general, Dr. Ben Karenzi, stressed that the government is not oblivious to the importance of nutrition in the fight against HIV/AIDS. However, he also underscored the huge challenge of maintaining an ongoing food support programme, particularly in the absence of adequate funding.

A woman living with AIDS cited in the same assessment highlighted this difficult reality. "They show us pictures of all the food we would love to eat, but we cannot eat pictures. . . . We have to have the means to purchase or produce the food. Visit us in our homes and see how we live. Then you will understand."

Rape Survivors

The experiences of Grace, Triphonie, Josiane and Didacienne attest to a critical need, not only for the availability of anti-retrovirals, but for more general support to enable the women to access the drugs. They were among some 200 rape victims who survived the genocide, many of whom were infected with HIV as a result, whose testimonies were included in a UNIFEM-funded report published by African Rights in 2004, *Broken Bodies, Torn Spirits.*

Ms. Rakiya Omaar, director of African Rights, told *Africa Renewal* that the most compelling issue that emerged from the the testimonies was not only women's dire need for anti-retrovirals and medication to treat opportunistic infections, but the difficulty in accessing them consistently.

"What became very clear to us was that even if the drugs were available, most of the women we interviewed were too poor to afford the food needed to take the drugs," she said. "If they did get some food they gave it to their children, as they couldn't eat when their children were hungry even if it was a matter of their own life. They also had no money for transport to the clinics. They worried incessantly about their horrendous living conditions, the desire to send their children to school. They were plagued by high levels of stress, not only for these reasons, but because they worried about their children when they were no longer around, which they knew was inevitable without ARVs."

What was especially painful to her, she added, was that a number of women cited in the report have already died. Every month she hears of more deaths, even though ARVs are now more available.

Little Grounds for Hope

Triphonie's story was typical. She grew thinner and sicker and her children went hungry as she tried to cope with living in a crowded, open army warehouse, rushing back and forth between her market stall and her four children to check on their safety. Her stall was rapidly failing, exacerbating the hunger.

Josiane lost four children to the *interahamwe*, the militia force that led the genocide. She has suffered debilitating memory loss. She was living in an unprotected shack without the means to pay for food or transport. Her 11-year-old daughter was a product of the rape and like her was living with AIDS. When her daughter got sick, Josiane would carry her to the hospital on her back. Although her CD-4 count called for them, doctors would not prescribe anti-retrovirals for Josiane because of her memory. "I was always confused," she told *Africa Renewal*. "I did not know the day of the week or the time of the day."

Grace, unable to support all four of her children, sent Juliette to boarding school. Juliette stopped taking her anti-retrovirals because she worried that her classmates would find out about her HIV status. Very ill, she was sent back to Butare. There she lay in hospital, unable to eat the hospital food, while Grace sobbed by her bedside, with no money to buy food Juliette could eat and frantically worrying about her three hungry children alone at home.

Didacienne would walk 10 kilometres to the nearest clinic when she was ill, a distance that, in her frail state, took her many, many hours. She could not afford the equivalent of US$0.60 for the bus that passed near her house on the outskirts of

> Without food and other related support, [anti-retrovirals] may not make a difference to mental and emotional health.

Cyangugu twice a week on market day. Not long before *Africa Renewal* interviewed her at her family homestead, she had spent weeks in the hospital. When she recovered and returned, she found that her small but well built house had been totally dismantled by her late husband's relatives. They explained that they thought she was going to die and therefore sold everything, including the bricks and roofing, to pay for the funeral. Didacienne and her children share a shed that housed the cooking hearth with one goat and a growing number of rabbits.

"Gift for Life"

These particular women have been fortunate. They have benefited from a small programme started by African Rights, called Gift for Life, that provides food and other basic necessities to women involved in the testimony project. The support is intended as a five-year bridge to self-sufficiency. Other organizations are also providing food to women in similar straits.

As a result, Triphonie has moved to secure living quarters minutes from the market and her stall is flourishing. Josiane's "permanent" memory loss is improving now that her stress levels are diminishing; she is taking anti-retrovirals and is planning a small business enterprise while her daughter, healthy on her anti-retrovirals, is attending a nearby school. Juliette was found a space in a local high school and Grace has found some work, and all live at home where there is enough food for all the family. Didacienne now has transport money to go on regular visits to the clinic to monitor her disease; she is getting stronger every day.

Anti-retrovirals generally make an enormous difference to physical health. But without food and other related support, they may not make a difference to mental and emotional health. Women who receive anti-retroviral therapy and food and who are able to cover the cost of transport to the clinics are finding they have the physical and emotional energy to turn their lives around. Most of the women in the African Rights programme, for instance, have opened bank accounts, a sign that they are planning for their future.

The UNIFEM assessment points out that when women living with AIDS are given food support to relieve their immediate hunger and to regain their energy, they then often request assistance for income-generating activities and skills to develop alternative livelihood strategies or to turn their failing enterprises around. "A combination of food availability and anti-retroviral therapy," says the report, can ensure that women living with AIDS "lead a productive life, become less burdensome on their families and communities and put less strain on the health system."

UNIFEM, in partnership with African Rights and with the encouragement of the Ministry of Health, has started an advocacy campaign to address the critical link between food and anti-retroviral therapy in Rwanda. The campaign regards treatment not only as a health issue, but as a critical path towards women's economic empowerment and self-confidence.

Triphonie, who was at risk of dying before African Rights came into her life, sat in the living room of her new home, her two youngest children eating with gusto out of a large bowl of nutritious rice and beans placed before them on the floor. She reflected on the changes in her life: "Only now am I able to no longer regret that I survived the genocide."

PILLS, FOOD AND SEEDS

Many health centres in Rwanda were finding that although they were providing ARVs to women who needed them, they were not getting the results they hoped for. The women visiting the clinics complained of extreme hunger and were disheartened by their inability to obtain the food they needed. And so seven clinics, funded by the US Agency for International Development and the International Centre for Tropical Agriculture, have begun an innovative programme. One of these, in Gitarama Province, has been particularly successful.

According to African Rights, the first step was to provide fortified SOSOMA (a nutritious mixture of sorghum, soya and maize) to the women to help them regain energy. The next step was to involve them in growing their own food crops. The project is based on the introduction of indigenous vegetables and tuberous seeds, which are well adapted to Rwanda's climate and soils. With this comes training in soil fertility, crop diversification and the use of hardy seeds.

To get women living with AIDS interested in the programme, Mr. Jean Gatsimbanyi Hodali, the coordinator, cultivated a demonstration plot next to the health centre. He encouraged the women to harvest the produce for their family's consumption during their visits to the centre. Then he distributed seeds to the women for planting in their home gardens, passing on tips and monitoring their progress. In order to join the project, the women were encouraged to form associations, known as amashyirahamwe. The project in Gitarama began with 50 women and soon grew to 90 as the results started to become evident.

Once the project was underway, the centre found that the health of the majority of the participants improved considerably. They gained weight, opportunistic infections have been reduced and in some cases the participants look healthier then people who are not HIV-positive. There is also a spin-off effect in the community. Community members in general have shown greater interest in acquiring the seeds and cultivating their own plots and the women in the programme have been encouraged to impart their new knowledge and skills to non-participants in their villages.

A Tale of Two Worlds

By Peter Gyves
America, November 20, 2006

In Sub-Saharan Africa, where antiretroviral therapy has increased more than eightfold since the end of 2003, great strides are being made in treating patients with H.I.V./AIDS. Those in the know, like participants in the 16th International AIDS Conference held last April in Toronto, Canada, express great optimism about treating the disease in the developing world. The United Nations' Global Fund, the U.S. president's Emergency Plan for AIDS Relief and the Bill and Melinda Gates Foundation have directed funds to this part of the world and made rapid progress possible. Although such optimism is largely justified, much work remains to be done, especially in preventing and treating H.I.V./AIDS in children.

Visiting African Hospitals

Over the past three years, I have visited Kenya, Chad, South Africa and Zambia to understand better the changes taking place in the care of people infected by H.I.V. What I have learned is that progress in preventing and treating the disease in children lags far behind the advances made in treating adults, and that among adults men fare significantly better than women.

During a recent visit to the university teaching hospital in Lusaka, the capital of Zambia, I met with staff physicians responsible for the care of children admitted with a variety of illnesses, including H.I.V./AIDS. I accompanied the chief pediatrician as she examined a child—H.I.V. positive, with severe anemia and malnutrition—and noticed another physician across the ward applying oxygen to an infant. By the time we approached this baby and her mother, the examining physician had just removed the oxygen from the child's face. The mother began to cry as a nurse wrapped the infant in a sheet and carried her away; her tiny daughter had died before much could be done to help her. The mother had brought her, in severe respiratory distress, to the hospital from an outlying clinic, because it had been unable to care for her baby. The examining physician told us that the infant was about 4 months old and appeared wasted. He thought it possible, even likely, that both the infant and her mother were H.I.V. positive and that the baby had died from an untreated AIDS-related pneumonia. Neither the mother's nor the infant's H.I.V. status was known.

This sad but familiar scenario, one I had seen several times before in visits to sub-Saharan Africa, was an unpleasant reminder that despite increased access to antiretroviral therapy in this part of the world, childhood death is frequently H.I.V.-related.

AIDS Devastation in Sub-Saharan Africa

The magnitude of the problem is striking. Since AIDS was first recognized in 1981, H.I.V. has infected 65 million people and killed 25 million of them. Today 38.6 million people live with H.I.V. Of these, 24.5 million—64 percent of the world's total—are in sub-Saharan Africa, an area that contains only 10 percent of the world's population.

Women and children suffer disproportionately. For example, 75 percent of all women with H.I.V. live in sub-Saharan Africa; they account for almost 60 percent of the adults living with the disease there. Despite this, only 6 percent of pregnant women in sub-Saharan Africa are offered treatment to prevent mother-to-child transmission of the virus. It is not surprising then that some 2 million children in the region live with H.I.V., which is almost 90 percent of the world's H.I.V.-infected children. Still, only 7 percent of the people receiving antiretroviral therapy in sub-Saharan Africa are children. Among the enormous consequences of H.I.V. infection in the region are an estimated 12 million orphans.

Mother-to-Child Transmission

The number of children with H.I.V. worldwide is directly linked to the number of pregnant women with the disease, and mother-to-child transmission is the most common way that children become infected. In the United States, the near universal access of pregnant women to a combination of antiretroviral therapy and intensive sur-

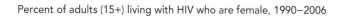

Percent of adults (15+) living with HIV who are female, 1990–2006

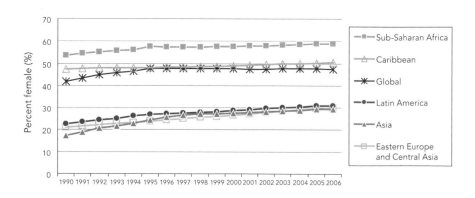

The United Nations is the author of the original material.

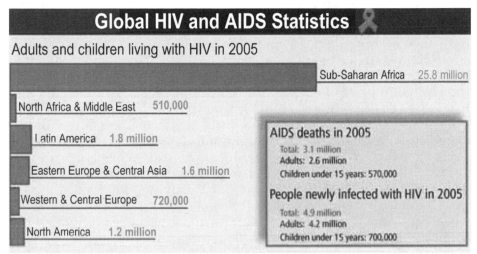

Source: World Health Organization © 2005 CNS

veillance of those treated has reduced the transmission rate to approximately 1 percent (down from 25 percent before antiretroviral therapy was provided).

What a contrast to the situation in sub-Saharan Africa, where access to such preventive programs is limited. Access varies from country to country and within countries and reflects the financial resources of a country, access to treatment centers of any kind, problems in identifying H.I.V.-positive pregnant women and varying levels of training among the health personnel who deliver and monitor the programs. Moreover, mother-to-child prevention programs in sub-Saharan Africa usually offer pregnant women a single dose of antiretroviral therapy at the onset of labor and one dose to the newborn within the first 72 hours of life. This strategy has decreased the mother-to-child transmission of H.I.V. from approximately 25 percent to 11 percent The simplified, shorter course of antiretroviral therapy is related to cost and the inherent difficulties in monitoring those receiving treatment.

Breast-feeding by H.I.V.-positive women is problematic. It increases the risk of transmitting the virus to babies by 5 to 15 percent over their first two years of life. Consequently, in sub-Saharan Africa the overall risk that mothers who have not received preventive treatment will transmit the virus to their newborns reaches 30 to 40 percent. Even the women benefitting from prevention therapy still incur a risk of some 15 to 25 percent. Despite the additional risk, the practice of breast feeding continues to be encouraged, because it protects against bacterial intestinal infections and ultimately carries less risk of death to H.I.V.-positive infants than do the alternatives: using formulas and solid foods during the early months of life.

A worldwide view of H.I.V. infection in children sees two very different worlds. While few infants with H.I.V. are currently being born in the United States, the number of infected infants born in sub-Saharan Africa remains alarmingly high. The nearly universal availability of programs to prevent mother-to-child transmission in the United States is further enhanced by physicians' ability to identify H.I.V.-positive infants quickly and to offer high-tech treatment Caregivers can quantify the amount of H.I.V. in the body, monitor drug levels to ensure a therapeutic effect, determine whether the virus is resistant to individual antiretroviral drugs and provide access to newer classes of antiretrovirals and antibiotics.

In sub-Saharan Africa, by contrast, identifying H.I.V. in infants is mostly limited to antibody testing, which often produces false positive results during the first 18 months of life because of interference from maternal antibodies. While treatment in this setting usually consists of a variation of the combination antiretroviral drugs used in the United States, surveillance remains a major obstacle. Issues range from the need to refrigerate some antiretroviral drugs to the prohibitive costs of high-tech laboratory testing and medicines.

Attainable Goals

U.S. standards for the prevention and treatment of children with H.I.V. are unrealistic for sub-Saharan Africa at the present time. Still, several attainable goals would significantly lower the prevalence of H.I.V. in children there and increase the survival time of children already infected. Here are some of them:

1. Increase dramatically the percentage of pregnant women enrolled in programs to prevent mother-to-child transmission (the current level is only 6 percent). These programs must also move toward the combination drug therapy and surveillance system offered in the United States.

2. Make the prevention and treatment of all women with H.I.V. a high priority.

3. Improve the general health care of H.I.V.-infected children, especially those under the age of 2. Improvement would include timely immunization against common childhood diseases and reducing the prevalence of malnutrition, tuberculosis and the most common causes of child deaths in the developing world— malaria and intestinal and respiratory diseases.

4. Provide care and monitoring for children who need combination antiretroviral therapy. That would entail a commitment to increase significantly the percentage of children receiving the therapy (from the current level of 7 percent) and a shift toward more high-tech treatment.

5. Encourage governments of the developed and developing worlds to respond to the plight of children with H.I.V. in sub-Saharan

Africa, allocating more H.I.V. funding for children and pregnant women.

Without progress in these areas, large numbers of children in sub-Saharan Africa will continue to be born with H.I.V. and to die long before their time. The current contrast demonstrates that the story of children with H.I.V./AIDS is a tale of two very different worlds. The achievement of the developed world in preventing and treating children with H.I.V. is arguably the greatest success story to date in the struggle to control AIDS, yet it stands as a tragedy alongside the number of children who are dying of the same disease in the developing world.

AIDS Orphans

By Oksana Kim
UN Chronicle, June/August 2004

It's called a "memory book"—a parent dying from AIDS jots down facts and prepares her child for the grim reality of a parentless future. Following case studies in psychosocial support for children affected by HIV/AIDS in the United Republic of Tanzania and Uganda, the memory book has been part of the best practices of the Joint United Nations Programme on HIV/AIDS (UNAIDS) in counselling children. In a sense, there should have been 11 million memory books in sub-Saharan Africa for the 11 million children orphaned by AIDS. And according to predictions in the World Health Organization's *The World Health Report* 2004, the number of double orphans—children who have lost both parents—in the region will nearly triple by 2010 due to the HIV/AIDS pandemic. Otherwise, the number of children losing both parents would have ideally declined if the 1990–2000 projections were to continue. Families, therefore, are under severe strain on account of the devastation caused by the disease. The developmental challenges of one of the poorest regions in the world now directly involve the future of 11 million orphaned by AIDS, out of 34 million orphans in the region.

"The world has never faced the prospect of tens of millions of orphan kids and societies so impoverished that it is difficult to absolve them," Stephen Lewis, the UN Secretary-General's Special Envoy of HIV/AIDS in Africa, emphasized. "It has been the most difficult dimension to respond to, because no one has ever encountered this phenomenon before." According to the *Report*, the number of orphan children could rise to 25 million under the age of eighteen by the year 2010. Mr. Lewis said: "It is a nightmare and it must be confronted."

Caught up in the circle of cause and effect of HIV/AIDS and harmed at both ends are women and children who suffer deeper implications than men. As women bear the brunt, children are left without any caretakers. According to *The World Health Report*, even though men and women are victims of AIDS in equal numbers, girls and women, who average 55 per cent of all people living with HIV/AIDS, are probably more susceptible to infection than men, due not just due to biological factors but more to "socially-defined gender differences." It further states that gender norms allow sexual freedom to men and encourage older men to take younger female sexual

THE IMPACT OF HIV/AIDS IN AFRICA

HIV prevalence among pregnant women attending antenatal clinics in areas of sub-Saharan Africa, 1997–2002

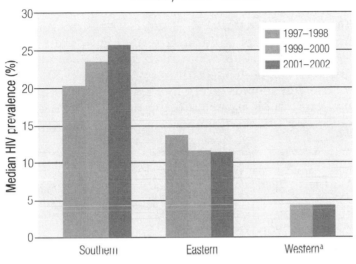

a No estimate available for 1997–1998.

Deaths from HIV/AIDS among health workers in Malawi, 1990–2000

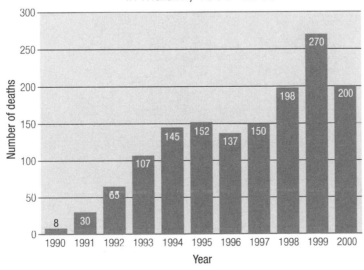

The United Nations is the author of the original material.

partners, while women are expected to be ignorant of their sexuality, bowing to socially-defined norms governing female behaviour. The *Report* moreover states that health-care systems expect women, who already do the majority of caretaking duties for the HIV-afflicted, to naturally fill such positions. It also warns that if preventive health measures tend to view the mother solely as a bearer of children and not as individuals deserving treatment, these measures "risk violating women's human rights and failing to attract as many participants as possible."

As entire generations of children are unable to grow into productive adults, countries in sub-Saharan Africa face economic collapse. The orphans have to be looked after by grandparents or extended families, whose households are expected to earn 31 per cent less than others. The problem seems to be not a lack of effective programmes but programmes of scale.

- No other region has been hard hit by HIV/AIDS as sub-Saharan Africa, which is home to nearly three quarters of the global population of people living with HIV/AIDS.
- By 2010, about half of all the orphans in sub-Saharan Africa will have become orphans because of HIV/AIDS.
- More than half of those orphaned by HIV/AIDS in sub-Saharan Africa are between the ages of 10 and 15.
- At the end of 2002, there were more than 29 million people in sub-Saharan Africa living iwth HIV/AIDS. Nearly 10 million of them were young people between the ages of 15 and 24; almost 3 million were children under the age of 15.

III.   NEGLECTED DISEASES

Editor's Introduction

Before HIV/AIDS emerged in sub-Saharan Africa, malaria and tuberculosis—not to mention myriad other tropical diseases, such as river blindness and dengue fever were considered the region's most deadly epidemiological threats. Though major strides were made against these diseases throughout the 20th century, some have lately experienced a troubling resurgence. Most notably, according to the World Health Organization (WHO), malaria is on the upswing, killing over one million people a year, and afflicting areas that previously had little history with the malady. While its reemergence has not been directly attributed to the considerable priority given to HIV/AIDS, malaria has nevertheless been identified as one of Africa's "neglected diseases," a moniker that applies to most major afflictions on the continent save for HIV/AIDS.

In this chapter's first article, "The Impact of Cultural Behaviors, Local Beliefs, and Practices on Emerging Parasitic Diseases in Tropical Africa," the authors describe a number of parasitic diseases that impact Africa and chronicle their various treatment methods. In order to better combat these maladies, they encourage the exploration of cultural traditions and how these practices can help or hinder modern health care, especially since many in the region are deprived of the benefits of mainstream progress due to "harsh economic circumstances."

The discussion of both ongoing and emerging diseases continues in the subsequent piece, "Africa Becoming Haven for New Diseases," by Scott Calvert and David Kohn, which explores the rise of new pathogens in Africa over the past several decades. Many diseases have surfaced in just the past 15 years. Calvert and Kohn believe that since most new diseases originate in the animal kingdom, and since expanding human populations are encroaching more and more on wildlife areas, new illnesses are likely to emerge with increasing frequency in the years ahead.

In her exploration of tuberculosis, "Necessary Treatments," Tina Rosenberg observes that three quarters of the world's population is infected with TB, but in most cases the disease remains latent. However, as a result of the immune deficiency caused by HIV/AIDS, people in sub-Saharan Africa are contracting symptomatic TB in ever-greater numbers. Rosenberg notes the many programs in place to deal with this burgeoning problem but also recognizes that greater resources are needed if the dilemma is to be adequately addressed.

The fourth and fifth articles explore malaria's impact on the sub-Saharan region. An editorial from the *Los Angeles Times*, entitled "Malaria: The Sting of Death," provides some startling global statistics: Each year the disease kills between 1 and 3 million people. Of these fatalities, 90 percent are African and most are children under the age of five. While organizations such as the

United Nations and the Global Fund to Fight AIDS, Tuberculosis, and Malaria are offering considerable aid to fight the spread of the disease, their contributions are nowhere near sufficient. In the subsequent piece, "The Exterminator," Kirsten Weir presents a controversial strategy for combating malaria. Up until the mid-20th century, malaria, a mosquito-borne illness, was a deadly fact of life throughout much of the world. However, thanks to the pesticide DDT, mosquito populations were eradicated, particularly in the United States, and malaria infections sharply declined. Unfortunately, DDT carried with it certain health and environmental risks and its use was subsequently outlawed. Weir believes, however, that the benefits of DDT use, particularly in regards to malaria, far outweigh its side effects and that it should be used to fight the disease once again.

In "Sight for Sore Eyes," James A. Zingeser presents an argument for the prevention of the spread of the bacterial infection trachoma. The article gives a brief history of the disease and focuses on how it is affecting the rural and impoverished populations of sub-Saharan Africa. Zingeser proposes that with minor preventative measures, much of the problem could be eliminated. If left unattended trachoma results in blindness, but Zingeser suggests that since the disease is preventable, teaching people, especially women and children (the most affected demographic), proper identification of symptoms and prevention will help curb an increase over the 6 million who are already blind due to infection.

The Impact of Cultural Behaviours, Local Beliefs, and Practices on Emerging Parasitic Diseases in Tropical Africa

By CELESTINE O. E. ONWULIRI, ET AL.
DIVERSE: ISSUES IN HIGHER EDUCATION, WINTER 2005

Introduction

According to the World Health Organization (WHO), health is not just the absence of diseases, but a state of physical, mental and social well being. People are sick because they are poor. They become poorer because they are sick, and sicker because they are poorer. Poverty is not just in terms of material possessions, but also in the realm of information. Lack of relevant information implies lack of knowledge. Similarly, inadequacy of relevant information implies inadequacy of knowledge. Having adequate knowledge on any particular matter does not automatically translate to belief, not to talk of practice. It is important that the right kind of knowledge is obtained, believed and practised for one to make an impact in primary health care, which is of paramount importance in the control and eradication of tropical diseases.

Culture, according to the Longman English Dictionary (2005) is "the customs, beliefs, art, music and all other products of human thought made by a particular group of people at a particular time." It further defines custom as "established and habitual practice, especially of a religious or social kind, that is typical of a particular group of people" (p. 336). On the other hand, the New Webster's dictionary (1997) defines customs as generally accepted practices or habits. If culture is the way people do things, then culture as well as local beliefs and practices influence disease patterns, incidences and prevalence positively or negatively.

Background

Parasites are found all over the world, but they find safe sanctuary in the warm climates of the tropics, which constitute the greatest threat to the health and socio-economic status of the people. The reason is that most of the infectious parasites complete their life cycles in invertebrate hosts. These, particularly the arthropod vectors, find the warm and humid tropics most favourable for rapid breeding and development. The high temperatures also reduce the duration of the developmental cycle of the parasites within their intermediate hosts. These two factors combine to ensure the production of more infective stages for dissemination to a wider range of victims. Also the tropics are ecologically less stable than the temperate zones, hence the ecological balance between man and his environment is easily upset by parasites and pests, thus making their effects more pronounced (Ukoli, 1990).

With the widespread occurrence of parasitic diseases, a problem of great magnitude confronts us in tropical Africa. The health profile in Africa is dominated by parasitic infectious diseases overshadowing the more fashionable conditions like heart diseases and cancer, which have assumed more prominence in the industrialized nations of the North; where most of the parasitic diseases have been eradicated or controlled (Ukoli, 1975). The modern approach to the management of parasitic infections, which involves the application of already available knowledge, includes the adoption of one or a combination of the following options:

(i) reduction of morbidity either

    (a) through chemotherapy or

    (b) by protection from infection and re-infection through chemoprophylaxis or immunization, and

(ii) reduction of transmission either by,

    (a) controlling the intermediate host or vector; or

    (b) controlling human behavior through health education.

These are the reasons why the adoption of the second options has not produced the desired results with most of the diseases in various parts of tropical Africa where they have been tried. The last option entails the initiation of certain actions aimed at modifying or changing certain attitudes, beliefs, local practices and behavioral attitudes which expose man to infection. The role of human behavior as a major factor in the transmission and distribution of communicable diseases had been recognized for centuries.

Nwoke (2000) defined endemic diseases as "infectious diseases present in a community in which the social circumstances do not offer any effective barrier to its [sic] spread" (p. 6). This reflects the important role played by social, anthropological, and economic factors in disease causation, transmission, and control. The pattern of transmission of emerging parasitic diseases in a cultural setting is regulated by a complex interplay of human factors including those which act as effective barriers to the spread of the disease and others that enhance its promotion. Therefore, a greater understanding of these factors is bound to help in determining what changes if introduced would upset the established culture-parasite relationship in favor of limiting the spread of the disease or bringing about a cessation in its transmission (Anosike, 1996; Anosike, Nwoke,

Dozie, Thorden, & Okere, 2004a; Dozie, Onwuliri, & Nwoke, 2004; Edungbola, 1990). To be sure, the results of such studies have so far not been widely utilized in the development of effective control strategies, particularly in tropical Africa where they are in their infancy.

Until very recently, the battle against emerging parasitic diseases through research has been conceived as a predominantly biological and biomedical enterprise. It is about time we harnessed the force of the "socio-medical group therapist" which encompasses those aspects of medical research that are focused on human behavior and its social, economic, cultural, and psychological determinants.

Many millions of people living in the tropics are cut off from the mainstream of social and economic progress by a combination of such harsh economic circumstance as poor nutrition, poor living conditions, poor environment, and a heavy burden of emerging parasitic diseases. Of 39.1 million deaths estimated by the World Bank to have occurred in these countries in 1990, 9.3 million were caused by infections of emerging parasitic diseases of which 926,000 were by the tropical cluster of African Trypanosomiasis, Chagas disease, Leishmaniasis, Schistosomiasis, and Onchocerciasis. Also respiratory infections accounted for 4 million deaths, while diarrhea diseases and measles caused 2.9 million and 1 million deaths respectively (World Bank, 1993; also see Nwoke, 2004; Ukaga, Dozie, & Nwoke 2000; WHO, 2004). The scourge of emerging diseases caused tremendous pain and suffering ranging from ulcers, internal organ damage, and disabling anemia to gross deformities of face and limb, blindness, brain damage and death.

Trachoma is the world's leading cause of preventable blindness. The World Health Organization (WHO) estimates that 15% of all blindness in the world is caused by Trachoma. Only cataracts cause more blindness worldwide but, unlike cataracts, Trachoma can be prevented through improvements in personal and environmental hygiene. Trachoma is a bacterial infection which is easily spread from person to person by houseflies. If a person suffers repeated infections over a period of years, scar tissue forms on the inside of their eyelids. The scar then contracts, causing the eyelashes to turn inward, often resulting in painful abrasion of the cornea and, in severe cases, untreatable blindness (The Carter Center, 2004). Today, almost all of the 146 million persons who suffer from Trachoma live in developing countries in Africa, the Middle East, and Asia.

Sleeping sickness or African Trypanosomiasis occurs in scattered foci throughout the Sub-Saharan tsetse belts of Africa, an area of some 10 million sq. km. About 25,000 cases occur annually in 36 countries in East, Central, West Africa and an estimated 50 million are at risk of being infected (WHO, 1989).

Malaria still remains the most important of the tropical diseases retarding economic development throughout the tropics. It is estimated that 267 million people are infected by malaria, with another

2.1 billion at risk in 103 countries (WHO, 1979). Currently, malaria accounts for about one million deaths annually in Africa, and it was estimated to have cost the continent a whopping 2 billion US dollars in 1997. Those who suffer most from malarial attacks are the impoverished, and malaria helps to keep them poor. The Roll Back Malaria (2004) year of 2000 showed estimates used to indicate that poor families in Africa spent as much as 25% of their annual income on prevention and treatment of malaria, with the consequent effect of slowed economic growth. The overall economic impact of malaria is seen in the slowing down of economic growth by 1.3% with the Gross Domestic Product (GDP) of affected countries being 37% lower than it would have been in the absence of malaria.

> Those who suffer most from malarial attacks are the impoverished, and malaria helps to keep them poor.

Schistosomiasis, also known as Bilharzia or Bilharziasis and caused by some species of flat worms (blood flukes), is known to afflict about 200 million people, with another 500 to 600 million at risk in 76 countries (WHO, 1990). Globally, of about 200 million people infected, 120 million are estimated to be symptomatic, with 20 million thought to suffer severe consequences of the infection. More than 80% of all these infected people live in sub Saharan Africa (WHO, 1990). In Nigeria, infection rates of between 1–50% have been described in the northern parts, 73–100% in the western parts and 32–55% in the eastern parts (Anosike, Njoku, Nwoke, Osagiede, & Okoro, 1998).

Ascariasis is the infection by the intestinal nematode (round worm) *Ascaris lumbricoides* which has a worldwide distribution. It is common in the tropics and subtropics, in places where environmental sanitation is inadequate. In 1995, WHO estimated that there were 250 million persons infected with *A. lumbricoides* and 60,000 persons died from it (Cheesbrough, 2000).

Hookworms are widespread in the tropics and subtropics. In 1995, WHO estimated that there were 151 million persons infected with hookworms and 65,000 deaths from hookworm disease. The two main human hookworms are *Necator americanus* more commonly found in the Far East, South Asia, Pacific Islands, Tropical Africa, Central and South America, and *Ancylostoma duodenale* found in the Middle East, countries around the Mediterranean, North China, North India, West Africa, South East Asia, the Pacific Islands and South America. The two hookworms occur together in West Africa, South East Asia, the Pacific Islands, and South America. However, the predominant species of hookworm in Nigeria is *N. americanus* and over 37% of the population is infected (Smyth 1996; Cheesbrough, 2000). Hookworm infection is spread by faecal pollution of the soil. Infection occurs by the direct penetration of the skin by the infective filariform larvae, especially when a person walks barefoot.

A. duodenale can also be transmitted by ingesting infective larvae. The total amount of blood lost to hookworms' infection worldwide is equal to that of the population of Togo.

Lymphatic filariasis (elephantiasis) is a debilitating and deforming disease condition caused by the filariid nematode parasites *Wuchereria bancrofi, Brugia malayi* and *B. timori*. The infection is transmitted from person to person by female *Culex, Aedes, Anopheles*, and *Mansonia* mosquitoes. The disease affects 120 million people in 73 endemic countries of Africa, Asia, the Western Pacific, and Latin America. More than 41 million of those cases are in Africa. An additional 900 million people are at risk (Anosike, Nwoke, Ajayi, Onwuliri, Okoro, Oku, & Asor, 2005). Lymphatic filariasis is ranked by the World Health Organization (WHO) as the second leading cause of permanent and long-term disability (The Carter Center, 2005; Lymphatic Filariasis Disease . . . 2005). The parasite lives in the victim's lymphatic system. In its severest form, lymphatic filariasis causes grotesque elephantiasis or dramatic swelling of limbs (usually the leg) and genitals (usually the scrotum). These conditions are devastating and affect the quality of life of those affected physically, emotionally, and economically. Chyluria is an uncommon complication of bancroftian filariasis which occurs when the lymphatic vessels linked to those that transport chyle from the intestine become blocked and rupture (Cheesbrough, 2000).

Filariasis affects the lives of a billion people mainly in Africa and Asia. Two types of filariasis are caused by the bites of parasitic infected mosquitoes and black flies. The WHO (1989) analysis estimates that 90 million people in 76 countries are affected by lymphatic filariasis and about 905 million are in direct risk in Africa, the Eastern Mediterranean, and Latin America (Abanobi & Anosike, 2000; Anosike, Onwuliri, & Onwuliri, 2003).

River blindness (Onchocerciasis) is caused by the nematode worm *Onchocerca volvolus* and is spread through the bite of a small, black fly (*Simulium damnosum*) that breeds in rapidly flowing rivers and streams along the most fertile banks. When a fly bites, millions of microfilariae are released into the bloodstream, causing incessant, debilitating itching. It is estimated that 17.5 million people are infected in sub Saharan Africa, with 270 thousand blind, 500 thousand severely visually impaired and 6 million having skin disease (Dozie *et al.*, 2004).

Onchocerciasis occurs in 30 countries of tropical Africa, south of the Sahara. Almost all (96%) of the estimated 122.9 million at risk of the disease globally live in sub-Saharan Africa and 17.5 million of the estimated 17.7 million who are infected live in Africa (WHO, 1995), while 326 thousand are already blinded by it (Anosike, Onwuliri, & Onwuliri, 2001).

Dracunculiasis or dracontiasis (Guinea worm disease) is an ancient debilitating disease caused by the nematode worm *Dracunculus medinensis*. Some authors claim that it was the "fiery serpent" mentioned in the Old Testament of the Bible. In 2000, a calcified guinea worm was extracted from a 3,000 year old Egyptian mummy (The Carter Center, 2004). Guinea worm or Dracunculiasis affects 10 to 48 million persons annually especially among adults of working age groups (Hopkins, 1998). In the recent past it has been included as a major devastating disease in the tropical countries (Anosike, Njoku, Nwoke, Ukaga, Okoro, & Amadi, 2000). The worst affected areas are in West Africa especially Benin, Ghana, Cote D'voire, Mali, Niger, Nigeria, Togo, and Burkina Faso (WHO, 1982).

A number of emerging infectious diseases naturally have been associated with the social and economic conditions of the rural communities particularly in tropical Africa. In these communities, the transmission of such infections may be related to cultural dietary habits (Udonsi, 1987) and usage patterns (Anosike *et al.*, 2004a).

Over the years, the communities, Local Government Areas (LGAs), States and Federal Government have in one way or the other shown tremendous concerns in the treatment, elimination, control or eradication of most tropical diseases such as Trachoma,

---

A number of emerging infectious diseases naturally have been associated with the social and economic conditions of the rural communities particularly in tropical Africa.

Sleeping sickness, malaria, Schistosomiasis, Ascariasis, Ancylostomiasis, Onchocerciasis, Lymphatic filariasis, Dracunculiasis, and others. Consequently, most of them are under some control, while many others are yet seriously emerging even while efforts are on ground to control them. Many of these emerging parasitic diseases persist in the environment due to several cultural practices, local beliefs, limitations, and even behavioral patterns.

Emerging and Re-Emerging Infectious Diseases

Fifty years ago many people believed the age-old battle of humans against infectious diseases was virtually over, with humankind the winners. The events of the past two decades have shown the foolhardiness of that position. At least a dozen "new" diseases have been identified (e.g., AIDS, legionnaire disease, and hantavirus pulmonary syndrome), and traditional diseases that appeared to be eradicated (e.g., malaria and tuberculosis) are resurging. Globally, infectious diseases remain the leading cause of death; they are the third leading cause of death in the United States of America. Clearly the battle has not been won, contrary to expectations.

Generally, emerging infectious diseases have been described as diseases that: (a) have not occurred in humans before (this type of emergence is difficult to establish and is probably rare); (b) have occurred previously but affected only small numbers of people in isolated places (AIDS and Ebola hemorrhagic fever are examples); or

(c) have occurred throughout human history but have only recently been recognized (gastric ulcers and parasitic diseases are examples). Overall, the emergence of many infectious diseases is related to environmental changes.

On the other hand, re-emerging infectious diseases are diseases that once were major health problems globally or in a particular country, and then declined dramatically, but are again becoming health problems for a significant proportion of the population (tuberculosis, malaria and many other parasitic diseases are examples). Many specialists in infectious diseases include re-emerging diseases as a subcategory of emerging diseases.

Impact of Cultural Practices on Emerging Parasitic Diseases

The role of food-handlers and vendors in the spread of faeco-oral parasitic diseases such as amoebiasis is epidemiological significant. In Nigeria as in many other developing countries, the selling of ready-cooked foods on the streets of towns and cities as well as in rural areas is now a common practice. It is important to point out here that cysts of *E. histolytica* remain viable for up to 5 minutes on the surface of the hand and for about 45 minutes under the fingernails (Beaver, Jung, & Cupp, 1984). In liquid foods (e.g., yoghurt, milk), the cysts may survive for as long as 15 days at 4°C (Nnochiri, 1975). The impact of this is that the involvement of these numerous food-handlers as vendors, with poor personal hygiene and dirty habits are conveying viable cysts to already cooked foods. Sandwiches and other foods consumed without further processing are very significant in introducing and disseminating amoebiasis and other parasitic infections. In fact, the habit of purchasing and consuming meals and snacks prepared outside the home is typical of the present lifestyle of some homes in Africa. The Food and Agriculture Organization (FAO, 1989) reported that 20% to 30% of the household expenditure in developing countries (including Nigeria) now is on street foods. And pathogenic microorganisms that are indicators of faecal contamination, such as *Entamoeba histolytica, Escherichia coli, Shigella* spp., *Staphylococcus aureus* and *Bacillus cereus* are frequently present. Therefore, street foods are potential causes of outbreaks of some of the notorious emerging parasitic diseases.

The habit of hand-feeding, which is a common practice by most Nigerians, especially in the rural areas may play an important role in the faecal-oral transmission of *E. histolytica* and related parasites. This is epidemiologically more significant in the rural and semi-urban communities where the filthy environment is "complexed" by poverty, ignorance and low standard of living. The use of hand-feeding of babies by housemaids and baby sitters (most of whom are brought from the rural villages), who themselves are riddled by a lack of knowledge and poor personal hygiene need not be over emphasized.

Direct faecal contamination of the environment is another significant cultural factor that predisposes our people to high incidence and prevalence of parasitic infections, especially amoe-biasis and enterobiasis. Such direct contamination may occur when premises or homes are grossly contaminated by the habit of indiscriminate defaecation, especially in families who live in crowded conditions with poor sanitation. This type of environment is typical of what occurs in squatter/urban periphery and refugee settlements. Furthermore, some practices in certain tropical countries, e.g., ablutions after defaecation, may increase the frequency of faecal contamination of hands and water and assist in the transmission of amoebiasis, enterobiosis (*Enterobius vermicularis*), ascariasis, and ancylostosomiasis.

Houseflies and other synanthropic flies come into contact both with substrata (such as faeces and other excreta, carcasses, garbage and other filthy matter) that may contain pathogens and then with human beings, their food and utensils. These

> The public health and economic impact of trachoma is enormous, doing harm to entire communities.

flies pick up and carry many pathogens (viruses, bacteria, protozoa cysts, ova or larvae of helminths) both externally and internally (in their crop and intestinal tract). As a result these flies are potential and often important agents of transmission of several enteric parasitic diseases (Curtis, 1998; Edungbola, 1990; Greenberg, 1971) including trachoma. In Nigeria, Anosike, Nwoke, Obiukwu, Nkem, and Nwoke, (2004b) and Dipeolu (1977) observed that such parasitic diseases that can be transmitted by these flies include amoebiasis and helminthic infections (e.g., hookworm, *Ascaris, Moniliformis moniliformis, Enterobius*, and *Trichuris*).

These flies breed in a variety of decaying, fermenting or rotting organic matter of plant and animal origin, dung, garbage, and wastes from food processing, sewage, and organic manure other than dung.

In Nigeria, transhumance (nomadic cattle rearing) commonly practised by the Fulani tribe is a great epidemiological factor in bovine Trypanosomiasis. The practice requires the movement of cattle and the herd's men from the tsetse-free zone in the north to the south in the dry season in search of greener pastures and water as well as the consumer markets. This brings the cattle in direct contact with the vectors (Anosike *et al.*, 2004b).

Since its discovery in Morocco, infantile Kala-azar has shown a slow but steady increase and the appearance of new foci of infection in various parts of the country. It is generally understood that dogs serve as a reservoir of the disease in children either through direct contact or as a constant source of infection for the vectors, *phylobotomine* insects (Braide, 2004; Ukoli, 1990).

The public health and economic impact of trachoma is enormous, doing harm to entire communities. More than 80% of farmers blinded from trachoma are unable to farm. Antibiotics are given to people at risk for blinding trachoma. Ordinarily, people are not supposed to be infected by this disease if only they could practice good personal hygiene and proper environmental sanitation. But what we see in many parts of rural and urban Nigeria is a far cry from the acceptable norm. In many parts, the practice of indiscriminate dumping of refuse and wastes of all types, which attract flies, is still very common. Children and even adults defaecate and urinate indiscriminately, worsening the problem. Simple maintenance of personal hygiene, observing sanitary practices and proper disposal of refuse and wastes will keep houseflies away and prevent trachoma. This of course will not cost any money, but how far have we complied? In the absence of compliance, many of our people are continually blinded unnecessarily due to this disease.

Due to poverty, as well as cultural limitations and practices, homes are crowded, people still build without provision of proper drainage, and open latrines still abound, both in rural and urban areas. These encourage the breeding of mosquitoes. Moreover, people still expose themselves to mosquito bites by not wearing protective clothing. Also, the practice of disposing cans, used tyres, cellophane bags, and other containers which retain water that mosquitoes can breed in is not encouraging. The practice of leaving heavy hedges around homes is unhealthy because these provide mosquitoes with hiding places. The old emphasis on cleanliness and proper ventilation of living rooms which is being forgotten today needs to be brought back.

The impact of cultural limitations in the transmission of Schistosomiasis is shown in the gathering of rural African women and their kids at the local source of water where they do their laundry, wash household utensils, draw water for domestic use and bathe, a custom which Wright (1971) considers as an essential part of the social activity of the village. Unfortunately the water bodies are ecologically suitable for the snail hosts of Schistosomiasis to live, thereby providing an ideal setting for transmission to occur. Equally of importance are the ritual ablution of certain religious groups before prayers and their custom of washing with water after defecation. In addition, some of the ablution basins have been found to be good habitats for the snails, thereby increasing the risk of infection.

In parts of Kenya the tribes' men have a custom of putting out their dead or dying relations for the hyena to consume. In Maasai land of Kenya, hyenas are heavily infected with adult *Diphyllobothrium* sp, while cases of the disease Paragonomiasis in man are not uncommon. In such settings, man serves as a suitable intermediate host for the effective transmission of the parasites to the hyena.

In the North West corner of Kenya is situated the Turkana district, which is believed to maintain the highest prevalence of hydatosis in the world. There are various hypotheses that have been suggested to account for the high prevalence of the disease. Among the human behaviour favoring the transmission of the Hydatid disease are the close relationship between the people and the numerous heavily infected dogs, and the use of dog faeces as medicaments or lubricants. Among other ways the dogs must have been infected by acquiring a parasite that is man-adapted and is from eating infected human corpses (Nelson, French, & Wood, 1982). Ordinarily, the development of the hydatid in man represents a dead-end in the domestic cycles of *Echinococcus granulosus*. A similar mechanism may be operating in the transmission of trichinosis in the sylvatic cycles in tropical Africa in which the hyenas are important.

Certain procedures in traditional medical practice promote disease transmission. In South Africa, some indigenous witch doctors prescribe ground-up concoctions of the proglotids of the Pork tapeworm, *Taenia solium* as treatment of tapeworm infection. Thus when taken by the patients the prevalence of cystercosis is increased (Nelson *et al.*, 1982).

The use of water for cleaning after defaecation and indiscriminate defaecation on pastures and around houses seemed an acceptable social behaviour in most rural areas of Africa. Here, communal feeding from a common bowl in the open street-yard (which is a symbol of comradeship) may also account for a high prevalence of soil-trans-

---

The environment, culture, and occupation of inhabitants of most rural communities have a significant impact on emerging parasitic infections.

---

mitted helminth parasites. Meals are often exposed to the wind, insects and domestic animals which may contaminate food with helminth ova while some participants in the communal dinner are awaited. As noted by Akogun (1989), the indifference of the Gumau people of Bauchi State to faeces, especially to those of children which are usually left exposed around houses a few metres from the dining place, causes diseases. Unlike the faeces of adults, which must be concealed behind the compound or in the fields, excrement of children is regarded as "pure" and is therefore treated with indifference. This cultural practice of most rural communities in Africa makes it difficult to control/prevent some of the emerging parasitic diseases.

The environment, culture, and occupation of inhabitants of most rural communities have a significant impact on emerging parasitic infections. The relationship between hookworm epidemiology and the ecology of the riverine coastal communities of the Niger Delta is of interest. The cultural practice of using hanging toilets over bodies of water (Udonsi, 1992) where human contact activities take place, in addition to the already contaminated surrounding soils, are responsible for the increased prevalence of disease among the farming and fishing population of the coastal areas of Niger Delta. In addition, the custom whereby traditional rulers must walk about barefooted (e.g., the *Obol lopol* in the Yakurr area of Cross River

State) encourages hookworm transmission. Unsanitary practices of passing out excreta indiscriminately sustain the transmission cycles of schistosomiasis, ascariasis, and hookworm infections. In many parts of Nigeria, people still believe haematuria has to do with male maturity (manhood signs). Among the *Tiv* of Benue State, it is regarded as the male equivalent of the female menstrual cycle and in parts of Ebonyi State, it is associated with irregular menstruation in women. In other areas of the East, people are ashamed of it because it is associated with promiscuity and sexually transmitted infections.

Guinea worm disease is contracted when stagnant water, contaminated with microscopic water fleas carrying infective larvae, is consumed. Victims often immerse their limbs in water, seeking relief from the burning sensation caused by emerging worms and thus recontaminating the drinking water (Onwuliri, 1982; Onwuliri, Obi, & Anosike, 1991). This is a harmful cultural practice.

When the Guinea worm eradication campaign started in Nigeria in 1988 the first nationwide active case search recorded 653,620 cases from 5,879 villages for the 1987/88 period. Three other yearly case searches were conducted, after which monthly surveillance began in 1992 and by the end of 2003, there were only 1,459 cases from 224 villages (The Carter Center, 2004; WHO, 2004). However, the first eradication target date was set for December 31,1995; it was missed and 16,375 cases remained recorded in 1,847 villages. The second target date of December 31, 2000 was also not met, as 7,868 cases were recorded in 907 villages. The trend was repeated in all six geopolitical zones of Nigeria. The question is "why were these target dates missed?"

Several factors made the realization of these dates impossible. Among these factors were the results of cultural behaviours, limitations, and practices. In the North East, North West, and parts of the North Central of Nigeria, the practice of ablution whereby water is used to rinse the mouth before prayers exposes people to Cyclops when the water is not filtered (Onwuliri, *et al.* 1991). This practice is also prevalent in parts of the South West. In some parts of the North East, it is believed that guinea worm disease is contracted when one has "cold blood." In the South East and South-South of Nigeria and parts of Benue State, cultural practices of having "sacred ponds" housing shrines and deities, which communities vehemently refuse to permit to be treated with Temephos (Abate®) larvicide, continue to remain "infection sites" for guinea worm disease (Onwuliri, Adeiyongo, & Anosike, 1990). Because people believe these ponds are sacred, they take water from them for religious and medicinal purposes without filtering them, in order not to "filter off the power."

The human immunodeficiency virus (HIV), the virus that causes the acquired immune deficiency syndrome (AIDS), was identified in 1983. As at the end of 2003, about 70 million people had been infected and more than 42 million still living with the virus while

15,000 people worldwide are infected each day. Sub-Saharan Africa is worst hit as more than 70% of the over 42 million persons infected worldwide live here and AIDS is now the leading cause of death in the region. Nigeria, the most populous country in Africa, has over 4 million persons living with HIV/AIDS and at the end of 2002 it had a national sero-prevalence rate of 5.8%; that shows an increase from the 5.1% rate of 2001 (Onwuliri, 2004; World Population Data, 2002).

Several factors have been identified as fueling the epidemic in Africa. Such factors include ignorance of the disease, lack of access to prevention, low socio-economic status of women, inadequate treatment and care services, and stigma and stigmatization (Onwuliri, 2004). It is rather unfortunate that even with the current level of awareness regarding HIV/AIDS, people still indulge in certain risky practices under the guise of culture and custom. Apart from unsafe sex, cultural practices like female genital cutting (nation-wide), local barbing with unsterilized sharp instruments, wife hospitality, wife sharing, wife-inheritance, widowhood practices like shaving the hair with unsterilized instruments, and "the spirit of the dead husband sleeping with the widow in the bush" (in parts of Enugu and Kogi States), pre-dispose people to HIV infection.

Impact of Local Beliefs on Emerging Parasitic Diseases

Differences in rates of taeniasis infection in rural Africa are related to variations in climatic conditions and ethnological factors such as human occupation, habits, behaviour, religion, and local beliefs. For instance, among the Goemai people of northern Nigeria, there is the general belief that roasted meat with traces of blood is a gastronomic delicacy (Dada, Adeiyongo, Anosike, Zaccheans, Okoye, & Oti, 1993). Some investigators claim that members of the *Maasai* and *Kikuyu* tribes of Kenya believe that consumption of measly beef guarantees their virility (Froyd, 1965) while the *Suk* women of Uganda are said to believe that it enhances their fertility (Bradley, 1976). Eating raw crabs for medicinal purposes around Okigwe, Umunneochi, and Arochukwu in eastern Nigeria as well as in the Upper Mango River in western Cameroun has been a major means of ingesting metacercariae of African *Paragonimus*.

The concept of blood in urine in urinary Schistosomiasis is interpreted variously by the traditional Nigerian society. For instance, among boys it is considered the male version of menstruation signifying the onset of puberty (Akogun, 1991; Okafor, 1984). While the Ezza people of northern Ebonyi state associate haematuria with coming of age, the Izzi people associate bloody urine with sexually transmitted diseases (Anosike, Okere, Nwoke, Nwosu, Tony-Njoku, & Oguwuike, 2003). Also among the ancient Egyptians, the prevention of Schistosomiasis is accomplished by covering of the tip of the penis with a metal cap.

In Onchocerciasis endemic foci of Bauchi State, Nigeria, adult males without scrotal enlargement are not locally regarded as "men." This is also the case in parts of Benue State. This belief emphasizes how uneducated these people are; hence scrotal enlargement is never associated with onchocercal infections (Anosike, 1992). Thus, enlargement of the scrotum due to Onchocerciasis is not seen as infection but rather as a mark of fertility. Such erroneous beliefs adversely affect the successful treatment of this disease, hence the issue of re-emergence.

In addition, nodules are believed to be due to hard work or overwork, accumulation of bad fluid, heredity, and witchcraft. Many still think dermatitis is due to witchcraft, enemies, evil spirits, contact with infected persons and poor hygiene. Some ascribe depigmentation to witchcraft, lymphoedema (limb and genital) to accumulation of bad fluid and adultery, and blindness to old age and heredity (Dozie et al., 2004). These lead to resistance to annual treatments by the Community Directed Distributors (CDDs). Further it is difficult to establish programs to control these diseases.

Furthermore, persons in endemic areas have raised speculations about the suspected negative effect of Mectizan on fertility. They believed initially that Mectizan, which was given free of charge, was an anti-fertility drug to check-mate increase in the African population. However, there is an opposite hypothesis. Evidence abounds now that Mectizan may have fertility restoring properties through probable reversal of early menopause in onchocerciasis infected women. Currently, men throughout the country seek out the drug because they believe it enhances libido. Anosike and Abanobi (1995) reported plausible reversal of secondary amenorrhea in three women infected with onchocerciasis due to Mectizan treatment in Imo State, Nigeria.

Ivermectin (Mectizan), a semi-synthetic macrocyclic lactone which has shown great promise as a potentially safe and effective microfilaricidal drug for the treatment of onchocerciasis also has a broad-spectrum deworming effect on various gastro-intestinal helminths (Abanobi, Anosike, & Edungbola, 1993). Presently, people from many of the villages indicated that the phenomenal expulsion of worms was the most remarkable thing about Mectizan.

Amongst several ethnic groups in parts of the Senegal River basin in the Republic of Mali, the ignorance of the people and their beliefs constitute effective barriers to their understanding of the nature of Onchocerciasis disease (Imperato & Sow, 1971). The popular belief is that the signs and symptoms of the disease which are the presence of the nodules, dermatitis, pruritis, and blindness are separate and unrelated and are, therefore, not manifestations of the same disease. Some believe that the nodules are a normal part of the anatomy or signs of aging, while the role of the black flies in the transmission of the disease is not well known, despite the discovery by Blacklock in 1926 that the *Simulium* flies transmit Onchocerciasis. Thus they hardly make any attempt to protect themselves against the bites of the flies, regarding them as nothing worse than a nuisance. Due to the high level of ignorance among the peasants of the nature of infectivity and immunity of the tropical diseases, they direct their efforts towards remedy by consulting oracles and witch doctors.

> Most people, especially in rural communities, remain unaware of the inter-relationship between water supply, sanitation and health.

Despite the efforts of the international drinking water supply and sanitation projects in Nigeria, most people, especially in rural communities, remain unaware of the inter-relationship between water supply, sanitation and health. This is because most cultures already have sets of beliefs regarding the causes of diseases. Such cultural beliefs are reflected in water and sanitation practices and contribute to the perpetuation of diseases such as dracunculiasis (Anosike, Nwoke, & Njoku, 2002). Examples abound in Nigeria in which villagers have continued to use traditional contaminated sources as their drinking water, despite the availability of a safe source. It has been observed that villagers used traditional water sources not because the traditional ones were more accessible, but because they preferred the taste of the contaminated water or because the pump broke down and could not be repaired immediately (Abolarin, 1981; Anosike *et al.*, 2004a; Onwuliri, Anosike, Nwoke, Okere, Asor, & Oku, 2005). In some other villages also, it has been observed (Nwoke 1990) that people believe that drinking pipe-borne water separates them from their gods. In some parts of northern Ebonyi State, (Anosike *et al.*, 2003) dracunculiasis transmission has continued after safe water has been made available and being used for drinking by villagers. Men in these villages continue to use the traditional, contaminated water sources in diluting palm wine (tapped around river banks) because they prefer the taste of wine diluted with the traditional water sources.

A similar practice in the etiology of Guinea worm or Dracunculiasis disease is shown by peasants' lack of knowledge on the relationship between drinking contaminated pond water now and suffering from Guinea worm disease twelve months later (Anosike *et al.*, 2003; 2004a). A survey conducted in some rural communities in Oyo State, Nigeria by Odiabo, Sobowale, and Ukoli, (1990) shows that up to 70% of the population claimed ignorance of the etiology of the disease. In the North Central state of Benue, people still cling to the belief that guinea worm disease come from enemies through "juju" and witchcraft, and therefore refuse intervention measures being put in place.

Conclusion

From an epidemiological perspective, many cultural practices, limitations, and local beliefs do negatively impact the emergence and re-emergence of parasitic diseases. This negative impact makes it very difficult for the judicious implementation of some of the new techniques necessary for the control, prevention, elimination or eradication of these parasitic diseases. However indiscriminate defecation, food and feeding habits, amenities and awareness of the mode of transmission as well as low levels of sanitation of most rural communities are among the principal factors promoting transmission of parasitic diseases. These conditions call for effective control measures in the rural areas. Perhaps, the conditions can be changed through community health education campaigns aimed at influencing the attitudes and behaviours of the population at risk regarding emerging parasitic diseases. Some of these cultural beliefs and practices are summarized in the appendix.

From the foregoing, the culture, local beliefs, and practices of a given population regarding emergence and re-emergence of some parasitic diseases should be embodied in any control, elimination or eradication programme for any parasitic disease. In this regard, the success recorded by the Community Directed Treatment with Ivermectin (CDTI) strategy of African Programme on Onchocerciasis Control (APOC) of the World Health Organization (WHO) in different parts of Africa is commended and hereby recommended.

Health education is a major factor in erasing negative beliefs of people towards programmes necessary for the prevention and control of emerging parasitic diseases. Once the hazards as well as the critical points for their control have been identified, health education can be designed to persuade the community and individuals to correct harmful and unhealthy local practices and culture, which increase the emergence of parasitic diseases in our environment.

Overall, since we know mat attitude is slow to form but difficult to stop, we must intensify efforts to change those aspects of our culture, beliefs, and practices that are instrumental in our exposure to parasites and other diseases. We must adopt participatory and interactive approaches in our relationships with people, especially with regard to control efforts directed towards eradication of any of the emerging and re-emerging infectious diseases.

References

Abanobi, O. C, & Anosike J. C. (2000). Control of Onchocerciasis in Nzerem Ikpem, Nigeria: Baseline prevalence and mass distribution of Ivermectin. *Public Health, 14,* 400–408.

Abanobi, O. C, Anosike J. C, & Edungbola, L. D. (1993). Observations on the deworming effect of Mectizan on gastrointestinal helminthes during Onchocerciasis mass treatment in Imo State, Nigeria. *The Nigerian Journal of Parasitology, 14,* 11–20.

Abolarin, M. O. (1981). Guinea worm infection in a Nigerian village. *Tropical and Geographical Medicine 33,* 83–88.

Akogun, O. B. (1989). Some social aspects of helminthiasis among the people of Gumau District, Bauchi state, Nigeria. *Journal of Tropical Medicine and Hygiene, 92,* 193–239.

Akogun, O. B. (1991) Urinary schistosomiasis and the coming of age in Nigeria. *Parasitology Today, 7,* 62.

Anosike, J. C. (1992). *Studies on filariasis in Bauchi State,* Nigeria. Unpublished master's thesis. University of Jos, Plateau State, Nigeria.

Anosike J. C. (1996). *Studies on filariasis in some local government areas of Bauchi State,* Nigeria. Unpublished doctoral thesis, University of Jos, Nigeria.

Anosike, J.C., & Abanobi, O. C. (1995). Resumption of menstruation in three women with secondary amenorrhoea after treatment with ivermectin. Annals of *Tropical Medicine Parasitology, 89*(6), 693–694.

Anosike, J. C, Njoku, A. J., Nwoke, B. E. B., Osagiede, U. R., & Okoro, O. U. (1998). Epidemiology of urinary schistosomiasis amongst the Izzi people of Ebonyi State, Nigeria. *International Journal of Environmental Health & Human Development, 1,* 6–15.

Anosike, J. C, Njoku, A. J., Nwoke, B. E. B., Ukaga, C. N., Okoro, O. U., & Amadi, A.N.C. (2000). The status of dracunculiasis in parts of Isieke Community in Ebonyi Local Government area of Ebonyi state, Nigeria. *Tropical Ecology, 41*(2), 183–193.

Anosike, J. C, Nwoke, B. E. B., Ajayi, E. G., Onwuliri, C. O. E., Okoro, O. U., Oku, E. E., & Asor, J. E. (2005). Lymphatic filariasis among the Ezza people of Ebonyi State, Eastern Nigeria. *Annals of Agricultural and Environmental Medicine, 26,* 98–204.

Anosike, J. C, Nwoke, B. E. B., Dozie, I. N. S., Thorden, U. A. R., & Okere, A. N. (2004a). Control of endemic dracunculiasis in Ebonyi State South East of Nigeria. *International Journal of Hygiene and Environmental Health, 206,* 591–596.

Anosike, J. C, Nwoke, B. E. B., & Njoku, A. J. (2002). The validity of haematuria in the community diagnosis of urinary schistosomiasis infection. *Journal of Helminthology, 75,* 223–225.

Anosike, J. C, Nwoke, B. E. B., Obiukwu, C. E., Nkem, B. I., & Nwoke, E. A. (2004b). Epidemiological implications of cockroaches and houseflies in the dissemination of diseases in the tropical rainforest zone of Southeastern Nigeria. *Annals of Agricultural and Environmental Medicine, 25,* 116–126.

Anosike, J. C, Okere, A. N., Nwoke, B. E. B., Nwosu, A. C, Tony-Njoku, E., & Oguwuike, T. U. (2003, June). Endemicity of vesical schistosomiasis in the Ebonyi Benue River valley. South Eastern Nigeria. International *Journal of Hygiene and Environmental Health, 206*(3), 205–210.

Anosike, J. C, Onwuliri, C. O. E., & Onwuliri, V. A. (2001). The prevalence, intensity and clinical manifestations of Onchocerca volvolus infection in Toro local government area of Bauchi State, Nigeria. *International Journal of Hygiene and Environmental Health, 203,* 459–464.

Anosike, J. C, Onwuliri, C. O. E., & Onwuliri, V. A. (2003). *Human filariasis in Dass Local Government area of Bauchi State Nigeria. Tropical Ecology, 44*(2), 1–11.

Beaver, R. C., Jung, R. C., & Cupp, E. N. (1984). *Clinical parasitology* (9th ed.). Philadelphia, PA: Lea and Febiger.

Bradley, A. K. (1976). Effects or Onchocerciasis on Settlement in the middle Hawal Valley, Nigeria. *Transactions of the Royal Society of Tropical Medicine and Hygiene, 70,* 225–229.

Braide, E. I. (2004). *Parasite, poverty and politics.* Twenty-second Inaugural lecture of the University of Calabar, Calabar, Nigeria, 36 pp.

The Carter Center. (2004). *Health fact sheet*, Atlanta, Georgia. Available http://www.cartercenter.org

The Carter Center. (2005). *Health programs*. Retrieved November 15, 2005 from http://www.cartercenter.org/healthprograms/healthpgm.htm

Cheesbrough, M. (2000). *District laboratory practice in tropical countries. Part 1.* New York, London: Cambridge University Press.

Curtis, C. (1998). The Medical Importance of domestic flies and their control. *Africa Health 25*, 14–15.

Dada, E. O., Adeiyongo, C. M., Anosike, J. C, Zaccheans, V. O., Okoye, S. N., & Oti, O. O. (1993). Observations on the epidemiology of human teaniasis amongst the Goemai tribe of northern Nigeria. *Applied Parasitology, 34*, 251–257.

Dipeolu, O. O. (1977) Field and laboratory investigations into the Musca species in the transmission of intestinal parasitic cysts and eggs in Nigeria. *Journal of Hygiene, Epidemiology, Microbiology, and Immunology, 21*, 209–215.

Dozie, I. N. S., Onwuliri, C. O. E, & Nwoke, B. E. B. (2004). Onchocerciasis in Imo State, Nigeria. Community knowledge and beliefs about transmission, treatment and prevention. *Public Health, 118*, 128–130.

Edungbola, L. D. (1990). Parasitologists and the challenges of the decades. *The Nigerian Journal of Parasitology, 9–11*, 1–2.

FAO. (1989). *Urban Food Consumption Patterns in Developing Countries.* FAO Rome.

Froyd, G. (1965). Bovine cysticercosis and human taeniasis in Kenya. *Journal of Parasitology, 45*, 491–496.

Greenberg, B. (1971). *Flies and diseases Vol. I: Ecology, classification and Biotic Associations.* Princeton, NJ: Princeton University Press.

Hopkins, D. R. (1998) Perspectives from the dracunculiasis eradication programme. *Bulletin of the World Health Organization, 76*, 38–41.

Imperato, P. J., & Sow, O. (1971). Incidence of and beliefs about onchocerciasis in the Senegal River Basin. *Tropical and Geographical Medicine, 23*(4), 385–389.

Longman Dictionary of English Language and Culture. (2005). Essex, England; Pearson Educational Limited.

Lymphatic Filariasis Disease—Carter Center Lymphatic Filariasis Elimination Program (2005, Nov. 21). Retrieved December 1, 2005 from http://www.cartercenter.org/search/viewindexdoc.asp

Nelson, G. S., French, C. M., & Wood, M. (1982). The background to the problem with hypotheses to account for the remarkably high prevalence of the disease in man. *Annals of Tropical Medicine and Parasitology, 76*(94), 425–437.

The New Webster's Dictionary of the English Language (International Edition). (1997). New York, NY: Lexicon Publications Inc.

Nnochiri, E. (1975). *Medical parasitology in the tropics*. London: Oxford University Press.

Nwoke, B. E. B. (1990). Cultural considerations in guinea worm eradication programme, *Africa Health, 12*(2), 32.

Nwoke, B. E. B. (2000). Ubanization and livestock handling and faming: The Public Health and Parasitological Implications. *The Nigerian Journal of Parasitology 22*(1 & 2), 121–128.

Nwoke, B. E. B. (2004). Our environment and emerging and re-emerging parasitic and infectious diseases. *Supreme publishers*, Owerri, Nigeria.

Odiabo, A. B., Sobowale, O. O., & Ukoli, F. M. A. (1990). Knowledge, attitude and practice in the management of guinea worm disease in two rural communities in Oyo State, Nigeria, *Mimeograph*, 12 pp.

Okafor, F. C. (1984). *The Ecophysiology and Biology of the Snail Hosts of Schistosoma haematobium with observations on the epidemiology of the disease in Anambra State, Nigeria*, Unpublished doctoral dissertation. University of Nigeria, Nsukka.

Onwuliri, C. O. E. (1982, September). *Endemic Dracontiasis in Plateau State of Nigeria. Its Epidemiology and Socio-Economic Impact*. Paper read at the 6th Annual Conference of the Nigerian Society of Parasitology, Jos, Nigeria.

Onwuliri, C. O. E., Adeiyongo, C. M., & Anosike, J. C. (1990). Guinea worm infections in Oju and Okpokwu local Government areas of Benue State Nigeria. *The Nigerian Journal of Parasitology, 9–11*, 21–26.

Onwuliri, C. O. E, Anosike, J. C, Nwoke, B. E. B., Okere, A. N., Asor, J. E. & Oku, E. E. (2005). Assessment of the effectiveness of intervention strategies in the control of endemic dracunculiasis in Ebonyi State, Nigeria. *International Journal of Natural and Applied Sciences 1*(2), 105–112.

Onwuliri, C. O. E., Obi, R. C. I., & Anosike, J. C. (1991). Observations on the ecology of Cyclops in Nigeria, *Tropical Ecology, 32*(2), 212–222.

Onwuliri, V. A. (2004, July-September). Total bilirubin, albumin, electrolytes and anion gap in HIV positive patients in Nigeria. *Journal of Medical Sciences, 4*, 214–220.

Roll Back Malaria. (2004). The Abuja Declaration on Roll Back Malaria in Africa, by African heads of state and government, 25 April 2000, Abuja, Nigeria.

Smyth, I. D. (1996). *Animal parasitology.* New York, London: Cambridge University Press.

Udonsi, J. K. (1987). Endemic paragonimus infection in upper Igwum Basin Nigeria. *Annals of Tropical Medicine and Parasitology, 8*(1), 57–62.

Udonsi, J. K. (1992). Human community ecology of urinary schistosomiasis in the Igwun River Basin of Nigeria. *Tropical Medicine and Parasitology 41*, 131-135.

Ukaga, C. N., Dozie, I. N. S., & Nwoke B. E. B. (2000). Reports of dissolution of nodules after repeated ivermectin (mectizan) treatment of onchocerciasis in southern Nigeria. *The Nigerian Journal of Parasitology, 21*, 39–44.

Ukoli, F. M. A. (1975). *Order amongst parasites.* Inaugural lecture, University of Ibadan, Ibadan, Nigeria. 42 pp.

Ukoli, F. M. A. (1990). *Introduction to parasitology in Tropical Africa.* Ibadan, Nigeria: Texflow Ltd.

WHO. (1979). *Epidemiology and control of schistosomiasis.* Report of a World Health Organization Expert Committee. World Health Organization Technical Report series 643, 64pp.

WHO. (1982). Dracunculus surveillance, *Weekly Epidemiology Records. 57 (9).* 65–67.

WHO. (1989). *Tropical diseases: Progress in International Research 1987–88.* TDR, Geneva, Switzerland.

WHO. (1990, March). *World Report on Tropical diseases.* World Health Organization Feature. No. 139, Geneva, Switzerland.

WHO. (1995). *Identification of high risk communities for schistosomiasis in Africa.* A multi-country study, Social and Economic Research Project Reports. TAR/SER/PRS/15. WHO. Geneva, Switzerland, 83 pp.

WHO. (2004). Dracunculiasis eradication. *Weekly Epidemiological Record, 19: 2004, 79:181–192. World Population Data Sheet.* (2002). Population reference bureau, Washington DC.World Bank. (1993). *World development report, 2984.* New York, NY: Oxford University Press.

World Bank. (1993). *World development report, 2984.* New York, NY: Oxford University Press.

Wright, C. A. (1971). *Flukes and snails.* London: George Allen and Unwin Ltd.

Footnote

1. Address correspondence to Jude C. Anosike, Department of Animal and Environmental Biology, Imo State University, Owerri, P.M.B. 2000 Imo State, Nigeria or at jc anosike@yahoo.com

The Impact of Cultural Behaviours

Appendix

Some Factors Involved in the Emergence and Re Emergence
of Some Selected Tropical Parasitic Diseases

Disease	Mode of transmission	Cultural practices, limitations, and beliefs that drive the infection
Trachoma	House flies (perching from infected to non-infected persons)	Indiscriminate dumping of refuse and wastes (inadequate environmental sanitation), not washing hands (poor personal hygiene)
Malaria	Female Anopheline mosquitoes (blood meals)	Poor drainage, indiscriminate disposing of cans, tyres and other containers (poor environmental sanitation), inadequate clothing, exposure of body (ignorance)
Schistosomiasis	*Bulinus* and *Biomphalaria* spp snails (shedding cercariae that penetrate the skin on contact with contaminated water)	Contact with cercariae-contaminated water, superstition (ignorance), indiscriminate defaecation and urination (poor personal hygiene)
Ascariasis	Oral ingestion of infective L_2 larvae	Not washing hands before eating (poor personal hygiene), consumption of contaminated soil, vegetables and fruits, use of untreated faeces for fertilizer (ignorance)
Hookworm infection	Direct penetration by L_3 larvae (*N. americanus*) and ingestion (A. duodenale)	Walking barefooted (ignorance), indiscriminate defaecation (poor environmental sanitation)
Lymphatic filariasis	Female *Culex, Aedes* and *Mansonia* spp mosquitoes (blood meals)	Conducive conditions for mosquito breeding (poor environmental sanitation), exposure of body parts (ignorance)
Guinea worm disease	Cyclops (drinking contaminated pond water)	Drinking contaminated water, superstition (ignorance)
HIV/AIDS	Sexual intercourse, contaminated blood, etc.	Poverty, ignorance, traditional and cultural practices, widowhood practices, wife hospitality, etc.

Necessary Treatments

By Tina Rosenberg
The New York Times, September 19, 2004

No one dies of AIDS. This is not denialism. The truth is that the AIDS virus does not kill you—it simply degrades your immune system so that something else does. Quite often that something is tuberculosis. TB is the leading AIDS-related killer, perhaps responsible for half of all AIDS-related deaths. In some parts of Africa, 75 percent of people with H.I.V. also have TB.

Tuberculosis is a wasting disease, usually of the lungs, and until the discovery of antibiotics, it affected millions of people even in wealthy nations. Today, more people die of it than ever—about two million per year—and in sub-Saharan Africa, cases are rising by 6 percent a year. The reason for the TB explosion is the spread of AIDS: having H.I.V. makes an individual vastly more susceptible to tuberculosis. In turn, TB has brought an especially early death to many AIDS victims. An H.I.V.-positive patient who contracts TB and does not receive treatment has a 90 to 95 percent chance of dying within a few months.

TB has played a part in making AIDS the plague it is today. But the horrifying collision of these two diseases also offers a double opportunity to save lives. The obstacle is that TB is still regarded as a relic. Granting tuberculosis the respect it deserves offers a crucial, and unheralded, way of delivering hope to AIDS sufferers.

In the long term, antiretroviral therapy must be made available to all who need it. But millions in the third world will die waiting. For many, curing their TB with a regimen of inexpensive pills or injections could allow them to live years longer. The very universality of TB makes it ripe for intervention. Fully one-third of the world's population is infected with TB. In the vast majority of people, the infection is latent. But when an individual becomes H.I.V.-positive, his or her immune system is less able to ward off the onset of active TB. So millions will suffer from TB early in the course of AIDS—sometimes years before they would have been stricken by another deadly infection. Curing this early TB can buy people years of health while they wait for antiretrovirals.

How many years? One answer comes from Cange, a village in central Haiti, where the Boston-based group Partners in Health runs a medical complex. In 2001, doctors from the organization published a paper about a group of TB patients they treated in 1994. They found that nearly all of the TB patients who also had H.I.V. were still alive in 2001 and that only 5 of the 27 they could track down needed to start antiretroviral therapy.

> In contrast to antiretrovirals, TB pills have the enormous advantage of being cheap.

Imagine a cancer drug that could bring patients seven more years of caring for their children, of working—of living. It would be considered a huge success. A drug that performed this feat for $11, in AIDS patients, without antiretrovirals, would be called a miracle.

In contrast to antiretrovirals, TB pills have the enormous advantage of being cheap: even though TB patients must take medicine for six to eight months, the complete course costs about $11. And the course is effective. Even the poorest countries can cure more than 90 percent of the TB cases they treat—if they employ a relatively new strategy.

That strategy is known as DOTS (Directly-Observed Treatment, Short-Course), and it is one of the world's most cost-effective health interventions. Malawi and other African countries pioneered the program in the 1980's, and in 1995 the World Health Organization introduced it globally. It is used far too little—in Africa, two-thirds of those with both H.I.V. and TB live in places where DOTS still hasn't arrived. But where it is used, it works. Peru and Vietnam cure more than 90 percent of their cases. Half of China uses it, and rates of cure there approach 96 percent for new cases.

A successful DOTS program requires a political commitment to sustained TB control. To prevent more lethal strains of the disease from spreading, a country must ensure an uninterrupted supply of drugs. Clinics must have a simple, cheap method of diagnosis and must track and report patients' progress. They must also find ways to ensure that patients take their medicine every day for at least the first two months. In many countries, the patient chooses a family member for this job. In Haiti, Partners in Health trains and pays largely illiterate community members as accompagnateurs. They visit three or four families a day, watch patients swallow pills and provide moral support.

Now suppose you are an African AIDS official struggling with questions like: How can I identify the sick and persuade them to come for treatment? How can I get them a steady supply of pills? How can I help them to take their medicine, day after day after day? If your country has DOTS, you already know the answers. You have a system that reliably gets drugs to patients, teaches them to take pills regularly and tracks their progress. And in many places, the patients with TB are essentially the same people who have H.I.V.

Doctors Without Borders has a pilot clinic in Khayelitsha, a slum outside Cape Town, South Africa, that combines TB and AIDS services. It started as separate next-door clinics, says Eric Goemaere, who runs the program, but doctors decided to merge the clinics when they noticed that patients were going out one door and in the other.

The fact that tuberculosis clinics are filled with H.I.V. sufferers should offer a way to solve one of the most vexing problems in both the prevention and treatment of AIDS—finding the sick and getting them testing and counseling. Yet less than 1 percent of TB patients worldwide get AIDS testing.

Why aren't more places adopting DOTS, testing TB patients and using their TB programs as models for treating AIDS? In large part, it's because TB is still invisible. The Global Fund to Fight AIDS, Tuberculosis and Malaria devoted only about 10 percent of its last round of grants to fighting TB. Research is so neglected that there have been no new drugs developed specifically for TB in the last 30 years.

At July's international AIDS conference in Bangkok, Nelson Mandela talked about the tuberculosis he suffered from in prison and the world's desperate need to fight the disease. "TB remains ignored," Mandela said. One reason is that he is practically the world's only famous TB patient since the Bronte sisters. It's a disease of the slums, of the poor and of prisoners. AIDS, by contrast, affects the rich as well. The sons of African presidents get AIDS. But they don't get TB.

And Mandela merely used to have TB. No one used to have AIDS, which is treatable but incurable. AIDS activists—without whom there would be no affordable AIDS treatment anywhere—are largely people who identify themselves as living with AIDS. TB has no citizen-activists—"People go quiet as soon as they are cured," says Alasdair Reid, who works on both diseases at the W.H.O. There are doctors who care passionately about TB, but they have been working in a ghetto. The world needs to join their battle—both to stop a tuberculosis explosion and to save lives in the fight against AIDS.

Malaria

The Sting of Death

Los Angeles Times, November 13, 2005

Over the short term, diseases such as the black plague and AIDS have killed more people than malaria. But medieval generations gradually built up resistance to the bubonic plague, and the discovery of antibiotics ended its deadly rampage. AIDS is a relatively young disease, a couple of decades old, and medical advancements are coming fast.

Malaria, by contrast, has stalked humanity since the beginning of history, reaping corpses beyond counting. It is a killer unlike any the world has known, a parasite that may have snuffed out more people since its origin than any other. And it's getting worse.

Malaria kills anywhere from 1 million to 3 million people a year, 90% of them in sub-Saharan Africa, most of them children under age 5. A study last year found that the child-mortality rate from malaria roughly doubled between 1990 and 2002, thanks largely to the parasite's growing resistance to older drugs and a breakdown in Africa's healthcare infrastructure. Every 30 seconds, or about the time it took to read this far, a child's heart is stilled by malaria.

Over the last six years, Africa's misery has become an international issue. Groups such as the United Nations and the World Health Organization have set concrete targets on reducing malaria by 2010 or 2015. Funding of anti-malaria initiatives has risen sharply. The good news culminated in President Bush's commitment in June to spend $1.2 billion over the next five years to fight the disease.

Yet nobody on the front lines is declaring victory. Future funding for Bush's malaria project is uncertain. The Global Fund to Fight AIDS, Tuberculosis and Malaria, the largest source of funding for anti-malaria efforts, raised less money in 2005 than 2004, and the outlook for the next two years isn't promising. The world is spending only about a tenth of what it would take to effectively fight the disease.

At this rate, none of these international goals for reducing malaria will be met. Millions more children will die, and a historic opportunity to crush one of mankind's most potent enemies will have been lost.

America Gets Serious

Last year, something surprising happened in the Senate: Key lawmakers began demanding answers from the US Agency for International Development about its malaria programs, a topic that had been widely ignored for years. Congressional hearings on the subject proved highly embarrassing for USAID; at one hearing, a former administrator had to admit that she couldn't account for how the agency had spent its $80-million malaria budget in 2004.

Finally, in December, USAID released a report breaking down its malaria allocations. The results pleased no one. Only $4 million, or 5% of the malaria budget, was being spent on proven interventions such as bed nets and anti-malarial drugs in other countries. The rest was going to U.S. consultants. Mostly, these consultants help African countries apply for grants from the Global Fund, though some also work on more concrete projects such as building a sustainable marketplace for bed nets in Africa.

During the 1990s, development assistance fell sharply, and USAID's existence was threatened. Instead of phasing it out, though, Congress transformed it into a contracting organization. Rather than giving money to foreign governments, it began giving money to American contractors. It formed a symbiotic relationship with these organizations: They would lobby Congress for more money on behalf of USAID, and USAID would distribute it to them. How they do it is anybody's guess. It is nearly impossible for outsiders to track whether USAID programs are effective, or even to tell how the money is spent.

USAID's report on its malaria funding didn't placate its Senate opponents, particularly because it was an extremely sloppy document, using only vague descriptions of project activities and numbers that didn't add up. Sen. Sam Brownback (R-Kan.) responded with a bill requiring USAID to spend a majority of its malaria money on concrete interventions such as pesticide spraying, bed nets and drugs, and to improve its transparency.

The bill never came to a vote, and it is languishing in the Senate. But it had an effect. Brownback, a powerful force in the social conservative movement, discussed malaria and USAID's shoddy record with Bush. A week before a Group of 8 meeting in July at which aid to Africa would be at the top of the agenda for the club of industrialized nations, Bush announced his $1.2-billion malaria initiative.

The plan seems designed to address the key criticisms of USAID. Dr. Ali Khan, acting chief of the malaria branch at the U.S. Centers for Disease Control, insists the majority of the money will pay for proven techniques rather than contractors, and that every dollar spent will be accounted for on a publicly accessible website. The $30 million needed for the first year of the project has already been approved by Congress, but the proposed funding will ratchet up later, and the initiative's future is unclear in the face of widening budget deficits.

THE AIDS-MALARIA CONNECTION

THE NEW YORK TIMES, DECEMBER 18, 2006

AIDS prevention has seen two breakthroughs this month. The big news is the protective value of circumcision. But there is another important finding: AIDS and malaria feed on each other, with disastrous effects.

In a paper published in the journal Science, researchers looked at health records from Kisumu, Kenya, a city of 200,000 with high levels of both diseases. They calculated that the interaction of the diseases increased AIDS cases by 8 percent and malaria by 13 percent. Over 25 years, that meant 8,500 additional AIDS cases and almost a million extra cases of malaria. The researchers drew on earlier findings that H.I.V.-positive people who get malaria experience a six- to eight-week spike in the level of the AIDS virus in their blood. During that spike, they are supercontagious, with double the usual chance of infecting a sexual partner. People with H.I.V. have also been proved more likely to catch malaria.

One important lesson of the study is that protecting H.I.V.-positive people from malaria would also limit the spread of AIDS. They need insecticide-treated bed nets to sleep under, and should take a daily dose of the antibiotic cotrimoxazole. Combining bed nets and cotrimoxazole with antiretroviral therapy reduced malaria cases in H.I.V.-positive people by 95 percent in one study. Cotrimoxazole is cheap, but is not yet widely used in poor countries.

The findings should add extra urgency to the fight against malaria, which has always lagged far behind AIDS in both money and attention. Last week President Bush convened a forum on malaria, but the fact that more than a million people—most of them under 5—die each year from a disease that is easily preventable and curable speaks volumes.

The study also sheds new light on why Africa's AIDS rates are so much higher than elsewhere: Africans' health is poor, and they are more likely to suffer from diseases—malaria, genital herpes and others—that make H.I.V. more transmissible.

Donors eager to fight AIDS have shown less interest in improving Africa's health systems, training health workers and equipping clinics. The biggest lesson of the new study is that it is all one fight.

Although the anti-malaria initiative sounds good on paper, it is still being administered by USAID; given the agency's lack of transparency and cozy relationships with contractors, that doesn't inspire much confidence. Malaria could be fought more effectively by giving the extra money to the Global Fund.

And the Global Fund could really use it.

A Visionary Program in Danger

The Global Fund to Fight AIDS, Tuberculosis and Malaria spends more to fight malaria than any other entity. Created by the G-8 and the United Nations in 2001, it has very low overhead and, unlike USAID, its spending records are thorough and easy to access. Global Fund money goes to pay for the treatments and programs that recipients most need, not what outside governments think they need. So far, about 31% of the money awarded by the Global Fund has gone to fight malaria, with the rest spent on programs to fight AIDS and tuberculosis.

One-third of the Global Fund's budget comes from the United States. In 2004, total world contributions to the fund came to $1.53 billion. This year, they dropped to $1.28 billion. The U.S. contribution dropped during that time to $352 million from $459 million. For 2006, Congress has already approved a $450-million donation, and a pending budget bill could add another $100 million. That still won't be nearly enough.

The Global Fund estimates it needs a combined $7.1 billion for 2006 and 2007 to keep existing projects alive and fund new ones. So far, not counting contributions from the U.S., it has only $3.7 billion in firm pledges from the rest of the world for those years.

Even if the Global Fund hits its goal for the next two years, the money spent fighting malaria worldwide won't come close to the amount needed. The World Health Organization estimates it would cost $3.2 billion per year to pay for all the bed nets, drugs and other interventions needed to meet international goals on reducing malaria. According to the Global Fund, last year the actual amount spent worldwide was $295 million. Amir Attaran, a professor of law and world health at the University of Ottawa who has written extensively on malaria funding, estimates that 2005 spending is less than $500 million. The numbers are equally bad for research on new products that could help eradicate the disease, such as a vaccine or cheaper, more effective drugs. A study released last month by the Malaria R&D Alliance found that the amount spent on malaria research in 2004 represented just 0.3% of total health-related R&D investment that year—yet malaria accounts for about 3.1% of the global disease burden. Thus, spending on research should be roughly 10 times higher.

Previous editorials in this series have described other measures that could potentially eradicate malaria but would boost the costs still more. An advance purchase commitment for a vaccine—a pool of money held out as an incentive for private industry to research cures for malaria, which otherwise is not a profitable pursuit— would cost about $4 billion. A global purchasing pool to subsidize the cost of malaria drugs for low-income Africans would cost $300 million to $500 million a year.

Not cheap, by any means. Yet far from impossible for a world motivated to stem the problem. In early November, for example, Bush proposed spending $7.1 billion on a program to protect Americans from a flu pandemic. Although there is a real threat of such a pandemic, it doesn't currently exist, and one might not ever strike the United States again. There's nothing theoretical about malaria or its victims.

The Cost of Doing Nothing

In 2002, during a U.N. summit in Monterrey, Mexico, leaders of wealthy nations committed to devote 0.7% of their national income to foreign aid by 2015. A handful of European countries have already reached this goal, and the rest of the European Union has strongly committed to getting there. The United States, meanwhile, has been reluctant even to admit it made the promise. Currently, the U.S. spends only 0.16% of national income on foreign aid, making it one of the biggest laggards among industrialized nations.

Given the economic and human devastation wrought by malaria, effectively fighting it would be well worth the multibillion-dollar price tag, which would only be a small portion of total foreign aid spending if the 0.7% commitment were met. Conquering malaria also would rank with walking on the moon and stemming polio as among the greatest achievements of the modern age.

The Exterminator

By Kirsten Weir
Current Science, November 5, 2004

Can an old pesticide that is banned in most countries defeat one of the world's worst diseases?

Few Americans ever give much thought to malaria. That wasn't always so. Malaria once infected—and killed—many people in the United States. During the Civil War, more than a million soldiers fell ill with the disease.

By the middle of the 20th century, malaria had been wiped out in the United States, Canada, and northern Europe. But it continues to be a serious health problem in many tropical countries. Malaria kills an estimated 2 million people every year, most of them children under age 5. Despite an international effort to control the disease, malaria rates in Africa have risen over the past few years. "It's going in the wrong direction!" said Roger Bate, the director of Africa Fighting Malaria, a nonprofit research and advocacy group.

Bate is one of several health officials now pushing for broader use of DDT (dichlorodiphenyltrichloroethane), a chemical that played an important role in kicking malaria out of the United States. They argue that DDT is the best option available for saving lives. But DDT is a touchy subject because it has been banned in the United States and many other countries for decades.

Bad Air

People once believed that breathing nasty swamp air caused malaria. In fact, the word malaria is Italian for "bad air."

Toward the end of the 19th century, scientists identified the true cause: a single-celled parasite they named Plasmodium. About the same time, scientists also discovered that mosquitoes act as vectors for the parasite, passing it on when they bite people. A vector is an organism that spreads disease-causing agents from host to host without harm to itself.

The malaria parasites need warm temperatures to develop inside mosquitoes, and the balmy southeastern United States was once hit hard by the disease. Malaria existed nearly everywhere mosquitoes did. During steamy summers, the disease reached as far north as Montreal.

Changes in living habits—a shift toward city living, better sanitation, and the use of window screens—were largely responsible for the eradication of malaria, but DDT also played a part.

DDT is an insecticide, a chemical that kills insects. In the 1930s and 1940s, when the U.S. government made a serious effort to wipe out malaria, DDT was one of its preferred weapons. It was sprayed on swamps and other wet areas where mosquitoes bred. Small amounts were also applied to some household walls in rural communities.

> Some scientists estimate that malaria has killed half of all the people who have ever lived.

By 1951, malaria was gone from the United States, but DDT was still used for other purposes. Huge quantities of it were sprayed by airplane on farmland to kill the insect pests that feasted on cotton and other crops. At first, no one worried about possible effects of the chemical on the environment. Then, in 1962, an ecologist named Rachel Carson captured the country's attention with her book *Silent Spring*, which detailed the dangers of DDT.

Carson described the damage done by DDT, which persisted in nature for years without breaking down. The chemical first built up in the tissues of fish. It then accumulated inside eagles and other birds of prey that ate the fish. It caused the birds' eggshells to become thin and brittle. The eggs cracked under their own weight, sending bird populations into a nosedive. The U.S. government responded by banning DDT in 1972.

Double Whammy

Many other countries followed suit, including a number of nations that relied on DDT for malaria control. A handful of malaria-ridden countries have continued to use DDT to control the disease. But even in those countries, DDT is no longer dumped in mass quantities onto the land. It is applied only to the inside walls of houses.

Because malaria mosquitoes bite after dusk, protecting people inside their homes can be very effective. DDT packs a double whammy: It repels most mosquitoes and kills those that get too close. It is by far the cheapest insecticide available and lasts twice as long as the alternatives.

South Africa was one nation that continued to use DDT after the United States banned the chemical. By 1996, South Africa had fewer than 10,000 annual malaria deaths. That year, the country switched from DDT to other insecticides. The new insecticides were also widely used in farming, and the overexposed mosquitoes quickly became resistant to the chemicals. By 2000, the number of deaths from malaria had risen to more than 60,000. At that point, South Africa turned back to DDT. Within three years, malaria infections dropped nearly to 1996 levels. In other countries where DDT has been used, from Ecuador to Sri Lanka, it has had similar positive effects.

Today, only about 20 countries use DDT for malaria control, according to Roger Bate. Many more could benefit, he says.

Public Fear

Why don't more countries use the powerful insecticide? "DDT probably has more opponents than any other insecticide because of its historic use," explained Bate. "But it's mistaking the point! All of the problems associated with it in the past are down to the mess that was made of it in farming."

Some wealthy countries worry about the double standard of supporting the use of a chemical abroad that they've banned at home. The memory of *Silent Spring* and dying bald eagles also lingers. Most of the money that tropical countries use to fight malaria comes from international donors. Many of those donors are reluctant to fund the use of a chemical that scares so many people.

"Why [DDT] can't be dealt with rationally, as you'd deal with any other insecticide, I don't know," Janet Hemingway, the director of the Liverpool School of Tropical Medicine, told *The New York Times*. "People get upset about DDT and merrily go and recommend an insecticide that is much more toxic."

Bate and many of his colleagues argue that the public's fear of DDT is unfounded. Billions of Americans were exposed to high amounts of DDT when it was used in agriculture, Bate said, without any harm to human health. And many scientists agree that the small amounts needed for malaria protection would likely have no significant effect on the environment.

Meanwhile, malaria is not going away. Some scientists estimate that malaria has killed half of all the people who have ever lived. Today, the disease claims two lives every minute. The most severely affected countries are in Africa, where the disease takes the life of one in every 20 children.

Some scientists worry that the situation could become even worse. As global warming heats up the planet, mosquitoes are spreading into areas where they once could not survive. Hotter temperatures also allow the Plasmodium parasite to develop faster inside the mosquito, infecting more people in a shorter amount of time.

Most scientists now think that eradicating malaria is impossible, given the complicated life cycle of the parasite. But chipping away at the disease is possible, and DDT has proved itself to be a valuable tool.

"The big picture is bad, but there are examples out there of what works," Bate said. "We need every tool in the arsenal!"

Seriously Sick

Malaria begins with flulike symptoms: fever, sweating, chills, headaches, muscle aches, and nausea. The symptoms come and go every 48 to 72 hours. Without treatment, the disease can get much worse. The parasites infect and destroy red blood cells, which can lead to severe anemia, a condition in which the concentration of red blood cells is too low to supply enough oxygen to the body's tissues. Infected blood cells can also clump together and stick to the body's blood vessels, blocking blood flow to the brain. The result is often blindness, brain damage, or death.

Drugs are available to treat malaria, though many are expensive. To be most effective, the drugs must be taken before the disease becomes severe. Poor families in places such as rural Africa often cannot afford the drugs, or they put off going for treatment until it's too late.

Some prophylactic, or preventive, medications are also available. When given to uninfected people, they attack the parasite if it ever gets into the body. But the prophylactic drugs are expensive and hard on the body. Travelers can safely take them for a few weeks or months, but the pills are too toxic for people living in malaria-affected countries to tolerate for long periods of time.

A Parasite's Cycle of Life

Malaria is an infectious disease caused by the single-celled parasite Plasmodium. The parasite is transmitted to humans by the bite of the female Anopheles mosquito. Plasmodium spends part of its complex life cycle in mosquitoes and part in humans.

1. A mosquito bites a person who is infected with malaria and picks up the Plasmodium parasite's gametes along with blood. Gametes are male and female reproductive cells, also known as sperm and eggs.

2. The Plasmodium gametes come together in the mosquito's digestive tract, forming a zygote, or fertilized cell.

3. The zygote develops into a cyst, or sac, and spores form inside it. A spore is a reproductive cell that can develop into a new organism without being fertilzed. The spores leave the cyst and travel to the mosquito's mouthparts.

4. The mosquito bites another person infecting him or her with Plasmodium spores.

5. The spores travel to the person's liver, where they multiply. The spores then break out of the liver cells and infect red blood cells. Most malaria drugs attack the parasite at this stage, destroying them in the blood cells before they can cause symptoms of the disease.

6. Spores reproduce inside red blood cells. Without treatment, the spores break out of the cells every 48 or 72 hours, causing recurrent symptoms, such as fever and chills. Some spores develop

into gametes, which are picked up by another mosquito, starting the cycle again.

Killer Genes

Scientists have tried for decades to develop a vaccine to prevent malaria, without success. Dozens of different species of mosquito carry the parasite inside them, infecting people with their blood-sucking bites. To complicate things further, four different Plasmodium parasites cause malaria in humans. Because so many different species of mosquito and parasite are involved, and because Plasmodium's life cycle is so complex, a vaccine has so far been impossible to produce.

Still, researchers haven't given up. Many are looking for solutions in modern biotechnology. In 2002, scientists sequenced the genomes of the most common malaria parasite, Plasmodium falciparum, and one of its most common carriers, the mosquito Anopheles gambiae. A genome is the total genetic information in an organism.

Theoretically, scientists could use that genetic knowledge to tinker with the genome of the mosquito to make its immune system kill the parasite. Or researchers could tweak the genome of the parasite itself to render it less infectious or less deadly. Such tasks would take years to accomplish, if they can be achieved at all. But the genomes offer one more target in the fight against malaria.

Sight for Sore Eyes

BY JAMES A. ZINGESER
NATURAL HISTORY, DECEMBER 2004/JANUARY 2005

A bright spot in an otherwise dismal prognosis for sub-Saharan Africa: Simple measures against trachoma, a bacterial infection that causes deformed eyelids, are saving the vision of millions.

News from the Republic of the Sudan seems to be relentlessly grim. Just one year ago, there was real hope that one of the world's longest-running civil wars was about to end. Negotiations between the Sudan People's Liberation Army and the Khartoum government were going well, and Ugandan rebels operating in the south, along the Uganda-Sudan border, were on the run. Then, in 2004, the peace talks stalled as a bloody conflict exploded in the Direr region, in the west; meanwhile the rebels continued their terrorist activities in the south. All of this in Africa's largest country, where the harsh environment—from the Sahara in the north to the tropical swamplands of the south—helps to lock millions of people in an infernal cycle of poverty and disease.

The vast majority of Sudanese live in a state of extreme deprivation and are terrorized by an appalling array of infectious maladies, most of which they are ill prepared to combat. Yet, they struggle on, and not without reason for hope: many diseases that have brought misery to millions for centuries turn out to be treatable and even preventable by the smart and dedicated application of modern medicine and public health.

Recently, in the heat and pounding rains of Malakal, a town in southeastern Sudan, a tall, elderly woman guided by a child approached a Sudan Trachoma Control Program team for help. The woman bore decorative facial scars—testimony of her Shilluk tribal heritage. She also bore other scars that testified to a life of poverty and neglect—the scars of trachoma. Both of her eyes were leathery and completely white, with no visible corneas or pupils. The program nurse gently spoke with her in Shilluk to explain that surgery might relieve some of her pain, but could not restore her vision. For this woman, the campaign to eliminate this blinding disease had arrived too late.

But blindness from trachoma is completely preventable, and the Sudan campaign brings hope that today's children may grow up free from such devastating effects.

Trachoma is an infection caused by certain strains of the bacterium Chlamydia trachomatis. The symptoms first appear as conjunctivitis, an inflammation of the conjunctiva, the layer of tissue that lines the inside of the eyelids and extends over the adjacent edges of the eyeball up to the margins of the cornea. In its earliest stage, most commonly seen in boys and girls under the age of ten, it looks at first like an unremarkable case of "pink eye." Close examination of the soft tissue inside the upper eyelids, however, reveals follicles—round whitish, pinhead-size aggregations of lymphoid cells that have gathered to fight off invading bacteria—that are characteristic of the disease.

That stage may lead to intense inflammatory trachoma, in which the conjunctiva becomes noticeably thickened, and small blood vessels within it become engorged, making it progressively redder. For reasons still unclear, as many as 10 percent of patients go on to develop severe, chronic stages of trachoma. With repeated bouts of infection, scars develop on the inner side of the eyelids, and as the

---

Trachoma can spell disaster to families or even entire communities in regions where trachoma is highly endemic, such as sub-Saharan Africa.

---

scars constrict, they pull inward on the skin around the margins of the eyelids. The constriction of the skin rotates the eyelashes progressively closer to the cornea. The condition in which the eyelashes are permanently turned inward, so that they actually touch the eyeball, is called trichiasis. When the in-turned lashes grate on the cornea, the trichiasis is painful and dangerous.

One obvious and traditional treatment is simply to pluck out the offending eyelashes. But that turns out to be a poor way to treat the problem, because it leads to short, broken eyelashes that are even more abrasive to the cornea. The body then "repairs" the damaged cornea with opaque scar tissue, which blocks light from entering the eye. If scarring blocks a substantial part of the pupil, the opening to the interior of the eye, the result is permanent blindness. Blindness from trachoma is not treatable, not even in the best of circumstances, because the tissue and blood supply around the cornea are so severely damaged that a corneal transplant would have a high risk of failure. As bad as that is, the blinded person still gets no relief from the pain, because the inturned eyelashes continue irritating the cornea.

Apart from being a personal tragedy, trachoma can spell disaster to families or even entire communities in regions where trachoma is highly endemic, such as sub-Saharan Africa. Children with impaired vision may not be able to attend school or do household chores. Sighted children are frequently needed as caretakers; in afflicted communities they are often seen guiding blind adults instead of attending school. Blinded adults can do only limited kinds of work; they can contribute little to farming or childrearing.

Trachoma is most widespread in sub-Saharan Africa, but it is also a serious problem in the Middle East, Central Asia, and Southeast Asia. Pockets of the disease also occur in impoverished areas of Latin America and even in Australia. Some 6 million persons have been blinded by trachoma, making it the world's leading cause of preventable blindness. The World Health Organization (WHO) estimates that some 150 million people are infected with the bacterium that causes the disease, and more than 500 million are at risk of infection.

Yet trachoma is a needless scourge. It is, at base, a disease of poverty and isolation, a disease of poor hygiene, poor sanitation, and lack of health-care services. One need not cure poverty to fight trachoma; it can be prevented largely through simple improvements in personal and environmental hygiene: helping people keep their chil-

---

[Trachoma] is, at base, a disease of poverty and isolation, a disease of poor hygiene, poor sanitation, and lack of health-care services.

---

dren's faces clean, and ridding the environment of the flies that cluster around people's eyes. Miracles can be accomplished with clean water, easily constructed latrines, and a reasonable level of community health care and education. The genus Chlamydia, which includes the trachoma bacterium, comprises bacteria whose reproductive strategy and small size at one time led people to consider them viruses. One species, C. psittaci, causes psittacosis (so-called parrot fever), a respiratory infection transmitted from birds to people. Another, C. pneumoniae, causes a kind of pneumonia. And C. trachomatis, in addition to including strains that cause trachoma, has other strains that are responsible for sexually transmitted cases of urethritis and epididymitis in men and cervicitis, urethritis, and pelvic inflammatory disease in women (the last is a leading cause of infertility in the industrialized world).

The strains of C. trachomatis that cause trachoma are passed from person to person through eye and nose secretions. The bacterium's strategy for spreading is a textbook example of successful adaptation. The irritation from inflammatory trachoma in children leads to copious secretions from the eyes and nose. Epidemiologicat studies suggest that children readily pass those secretions to family members and peers in many simple, insidious ways, such as on fingers, clothes, shared bedding and towels. Eye and nose secretions also attract moisture-seeking flies, which appear to transmit the bacteria as well.

Consistent with these means of transmission, trachoma is primarily a disease of women and children. In most populations women are as much as three times more likely to develop trichiasis than men are. Most public health experts believe the reason for the imbalance is that women are the primary caregivers of children and are therefore reinfected repeatedly.

Trachoma was described as a clinical disease thousands of years before the bacterium was first isolated and identified. An illness resembling trachoma appears in a compilation of Chinese medical texts probably written down in their present form at least two millennia ago and traditionally believed to date from the time of the Emperor Huang Ti (the twenty-seventh century B.C.). The Ebers Papyrus from Egypt, dating from about 1550 B.C., includes prescriptions for trachoma. In ancient tombs Egyptologists have discovered what were probably tools for treating trachoma by plucking eyelashes. Evidence of trachoma has even been found in mummies.

In later antiquity many important Greek physicians, including Hippocrates and Galen, refer to trachoma and its treatment in their writings. The first record of the word trachoma is attributed to Dioscorides in A.D. 60; the term derives from the Greek for "rough eye," an apt description. From the eighth until the fourteenth centuries A.D., Arab ophthalmologists were the primary source of information on trachoma. They understood that the disease was contagious and distinguished between acute and chronic stages.

Soldiers in the Napoleonic campaigns of 1798 through 1802 encountered trachoma in Egypt, where it was called "military," or "Egyptian" ophthalmia. On their return they brought it to western Europe, where its spread was fueled by the crowded and unhygienic urban conditions fostered by the Industrial Revolution. In 1805, in response to a huge epidemic of Egyptian ophthalmia, the surgeon John Cunningham Saunders founded the London Dispensary for Curing Diseases of the Eye and Ear, the world's first specialist eye hospital.

Across the Atlantic, trachoma proved to be such an important public health concern that in the late nineteenth and early twentieth centuries, U.S. immigration officials refused entry to people suspected of having the disease. With improvements in hygiene and sanitation, trachoma disappeared from U.S. cities, and by the late 1950s, the last of the nation's trachoma hospitals had closed their doors or had been converted into general eye hospitals. Nevertheless, pockets of trachoma continued to exist even into the 1960s, particularly in impoverished Native American communities of the Southwest.

The transmission and ecology of the disease have dictated the priorities of the public health community: to develop strategies for controlling the disease in underdeveloped and underserved populations. In 1987 WHO recommended simplified standards for assessing trachoma infection, so that examinations could be performed not only by ophthalmologists but also by nurses and other healthcare workers using widely available instruments (a portable light source and magnifying lens). The WHO protocol thus made it possible to survey the geographic extent and severity of the disease.

A turning point came in 1996, when the Edna McConnell Clark Foundation, based in New York City, sponsored a meeting at WHO headquarters, bringing health professionals, medical researchers, and philanthropic donors together. The result was a concrete plan for eliminating blindness caused by trachoma, with a strategy applicable in every village in the world, no matter how poor or how isolated. The strategy was called "SAFE"—an acronym for surgery (to correct trichiasis), antibiotics (to treat inflammatory trachoma and reduce C. trachoma in the environment), facial cleanliness, and environmental improvement (to prevent transmission of trachoma).

The surgery is a simple procedure for realigning the inturned eyelashes of trichiasis patients. It can be done by nurses in village health centers or anywhere else (a classroom, for instance) that can be cleaned and properly equipped.

Antibiotics provide a second line of attack. Throughout the 1980s the standard treatment was to apply tetracycline ointment topically on the eyes twice a day for six weeks. But the treatment, besides being lengthy, was messy and uncomfortable; its success was only limited. Subsequent research on the antibiotic azithromycin showed that a single oral dose of the drug is as effective as six weeks of the topical therapy. In November 1998, the pharmaceutical company Pfizer Inc., based in New York City, in collaboration with the Clark Foundation, launched the International Trachoma Initiative to manage a long-term donation of Zithromax, Pfizer's brand of azithromycin.

To further promote trachoma control, WHO created a new working group, the Alliance for the Global Elimination of Blinding Trachoma by the Year 2020 (known by the acronym "GET 2020"), which held its first meeting in 1997. Early on, the alliance recognized that none of its partners was committed primarily to supporting the improvement of local hygiene, the F and E of the SAFE strategy. One of the alliance members approached the Carter Center, founded by former president Jimmy Carter and his wife Rosalynn Carter, to help in that role. My affiliation with the Carter Center led to my own participation in the project.

The Carter Center had already demonstrated its ability to manage a similar effort, coordinating a successful program to reduce the incidence of guinea worm disease, primarily in sub-Saharan Africa. As its name implies, that illness is caused by a parasite; it is transmitted solely through infected drinking water. For my colleagues and me at the Carter Center, joining the alliance actually offered a solution to a dilemma: how to redirect the efforts of the workers and volunteers, whose progress in combating guinea worm disease was (happily) threatening to leave them without a job to do. In 1998 and

1999, the Carter Center began working with governments and partner organizations in Ethiopia, Ghana, Mali, Niger, Nigeria, Sudan, and Yemen to control trachoma.

The first step in combating trachoma is to survey the extent and severity of disease where it is endemic. Such baseline studies can yield surprising results. For example, it had long been assumed that in arid, dusty environments, the irritation to people's eyes due to the dryness and dust would increase the risk of transmitting the bacterium. In Sudan, however, there proved to be high levels of infection both around Wadi Halfa, a desert settlement on the nation's northern border, and around Malakal, a town in the humid, lush south. One of the most disturbing findings in the Malakal area was that children as young as five years old were afflicted with trichiasis.

Epidemiological surveys are fine for measuring the prevalence of a disease, or the relative importance of risk factors such as age and lack of access to clean water. But such baseline data do not necessarily show why the risk factors exist—or how to change them. Why, for instance, aren't children's faces kept clean? (Some tribes think washing children's faces is unhealthy.) Why are there no latrines— or, if there are, is there some cultural reason they are not used or maintained? (In southern Sudan, the soil is waterlogged and latrines collapse.) What do people think causes the disease? (We found that some people believe trachoma can be caught by looking at the eyes of someone who is infected with the disease.) To seek answers to such questions, the Carter Center made sociological surveys in Ghana in 1999 and in the South Gondar zone of northern Ethiopia in 2001.

A related cultural concern we had was to identify the best channels for communicating with a particular community. In Ghana, for instance, the popular medium of radio is so cost-effective in reaching isolated rural areas that most trachoma control programs provide financial and technical support for radio programming and short broadcast messages. Program supervisors, however, reported that villagers who had heard jingles and radio spots about trachoma control often did not understand the content of the messages. In response, the Ghanaian trachoma control workers organized radio listening clubs, each with about twenty-five members. Each club is given a windup radio, and the club members meet to listen to broadcasts about trachoma control and then discuss them. Guided by a facilitator, club members begin by learning the jingles and slogans by rote, and then move on to translating the messages into sustainable community changes.

Cultural understanding is not the only approach to trachoma control. Where flies are a problem, for instance, an effective measure is to eliminate fly-breeding sites, such as human feces left uncovered on the ground. In 2002 Niger's National Blindness Prevention Program and the Carter Center began promoting latrine construction in the country's Zinder region, where trachoma is well entrenched.

Each village and household that would benefit from a new latrine supplied much of the labor and materials for digging it and building its enclosure. The local economy also paid local masons for their work. The only things supplied by the national program were training for the masons, and the tools, cement, and iron rebar for their work. By the end of the year, 1,282 latrines had been completed by such community-based projects.

The latrine program also included community-based (as opposed to school- or clinic-based) education to promote regular face and hand washing and more frequent washing of clothes and towels. Not surprisingly, the demand for soap grew, but that led to a new problem: commercial soaps in the Zinder region are expensive and, often, not even available.

The solution was to revive the neglected craft of soap making. Early in 2003, the first group of thirty women from ten villages in rural Zinder got a two-day training session in the traditional production of soap. The women learned how to make soap from readily available materials: soda (made by filtering ashes through water), animal or plant oil, and water. The mixture is heated over a low fire, then formed into shape and cooled. Soap made this way is affordable in the poorest of villages, and it can even be sold to generate outside income.

While prevention and hygiene are being pursued, those who already suffer from trachoma must be treated as well: the S (for surgery) and A (for antibiotics) are essential tools of the overall strategy. In 2002, in the South Gondar Zone of Ethiopia, the Amhara Health Bureau trained nineteen surgeons in the treatment of trichiasis and supplied them with a hundred new surgical kits. From 2002 through 2003, a total of more than 10,000 trichiasis patients received corrective surgery—a healthy number, but still less than 30 percent of the estimated backlog of patients needing surgery in that zone.

As for antibiotics, even the war zones of southern Sudan show cause for hope. In both opposition- and government-controlled areas, as well as in camps for internally displaced persons near Khartoum, nearly 200,000 Sudanese were treated with azithromycin in 2002. To do so, health workers sometimes had to undertake "hit-and-run" treatment campaigns to avoid being caught in combat. Still, according to a follow-up survey made that same year, all the villages that had implemented the SAFE strategy for at least two years underwent a statistically significant drop in the prevalence of trachoma infection among children.

Dedicated health workers from the government of Sudan and Sudanese health-care workers in nongovernmental organizations (NGOs) continue to promote the SAFE strategy in some of the most isolated and impoverished places in the world. In 2003, one NGO working in western Darfur was forced to abandon trachoma control activities when fighting erupted there. In 2004, two NGOs working near Malakal were evacuated owing to mounting insecurity. And yet the program continues to expand and improve. This past September, teams from the Sudan Trachoma Control Program in both the north and south reported they were on track to deliver more than 680,000 azithromycin treatments in 2004 to people at risk for the blinding effects of trachoma, proof that not all the news from Sudan is grim.

The ultimate goal of the SAFE strategy is to eliminate the threat of blindness caused by trachoma by the year 2020. Meeting that goal alone would save millions from untold misery, but it would also bring enormous side benefits. Improved personal and environmental hygiene could have a substantial positive impact on diarrheal, respiratory, and several parasitic diseases. Nurses and eye-care workers who have sharpened their skills with the training needed to do eyelid surgery would improve the general quality of eye care and health services. Most important of all, demonstrating to villagers that they can take charge of bettering their own health and lives can give them the hope they need to break the cycle of poverty and disease once and for all.

IV. Problems and Solutions for African Health Care Systems

Editor's Introduction

Not only is sub-Saharan Africa an amalgam of disparate cultures, but it is also still affected by the remnants of colonization, which include social and governmental structures. This mixture creates difficulties for those who are attempting to improve the state of health care on the continent. With politicians serving their own agendas, rampant poverty, recurring famine and war, and problems with communication due either to geography, culture, or language, a variety of solutions have been proposed.

In the chapter's first article, "'Brain drain' Puts Africa's Hospitals on the Critical List," Andrew Jack for the London *Financial Times* delves into the biggest problem facing the health care system in modern-day Africa. In a recent report by the World Health Organization, it was shown that numerous health-care workers are migrating to richer countries because salaries in Africa are extremely low. With the smallest ratio of health care professionals to patients, the quality of care in sub-Saharan Africa is suffering. This is especially true for one of Africa's poorest nations, Malawi, where 12 million people are served by only 100 doctors and 2,000 nurses. In the second article, "Botswana Health Care System Needs Dialogue," Dr. Vincent Molelekwa describes conditions in one particular country and explains how it is fighting to keep its nurses and doctors within its borders. Nevertheless, with the cost of training outweighing salaries for these professionals, the Diaspora continues unabated.

One way of improving the health care system is by creating an amalgamation of all available resources, and many countries are beginning to realize that relying on public health care alone is ineffective, especially when it comes to treating rural populations. In the chapter's third article, "Private Sector, Human Resources and Health Franchising in Africa," a report prepared by Ndola Prata, Dominic Montagu, and Emma Jefferys for the World Health Organization, the writers support the inclusion of private health care systems and health franchising into the already established public system, because health spending is currently not reaching the poor.

Alongside the introduction of private enterprise into the health care system, many in Africa are calling for closer relationships with practitioners of traditional African medicine. Both the fourth and fifth articles claim that by incorporating tradition healers into the health care system the advantages would be enormous. In "Defining Minimum Standards of Practice for Incorporating African Traditional Medicine into HIV/AIDS Prevention, Care, and Support," Jaco Homsy suggests that one of the most important factors in this awareness is that a high percentage of the sub-Saharan population obtains medical advice from traditional healers, and that the combination of modern and traditional health care would reach a greater portion of the populace. In "*Sango-*

mas Step out of the Shadows," Tom Nevin furthers this discussion by also suggesting the need to bridge the gap between traditional and bio-medicine. He recognizes that there is much to be learned about this potential collaboration, but since $65 billion are spent on traditional medicine each year, he believes it would be worth the time and money to investigate such a partnership further.

"Brain drain" Puts Africa's Hospitals on the Critical List

By Andrew Jack
Financial Times, July 7, 2005

The recently completed district hospital in Thyolo in southern Malawi would not look out of place in a more developed country except for one thing—a chronic shortage of medical staff.

The building—built with the support of the European Union—houses just 40 overworked nurses and eight clinical staff. It has no full-time doctor.

In the whole of Malawi, a country of 12m people, there are just 100 doctors and 2,000 nurses.

Malawi, one of the world's poorest countries, has always struggled to train the medical staff it needs. But now its plight has been exacerbated by a brain drain as staff are lured abroad by the prospect of higher pay in developed countries.

As the leaders of the Group of Eight industrialised nations meet in Gleneagles, Scotland, this week to discuss African poverty, Malawi's struggle to provide basic healthcare for its people offers a stark reminder to the world's richest countries that they contribute to the problems that many African nations face.

"Taking people away to other health services is killing our people," says Dr Hetherwick Ntabe, Malawi's health minister. He sees little hope of any solution in the near term.

Dr Atta Gbary, the World Health Organisation's Africa adviser on human resources in health, estimates that 23,000 of the best trained medical staff leave Africa each year for the developed world. He says that there are just 800,000 medical staff in the whole of Africa.

Given that the cost of training a specialist doctor in Africa is estimated by the United Nations to be about Dollars 100,000, the exodus represents a Dollars 500m annual subsidy from Africa to wealthy nations. In the UK last year there were more than 10,200 African-trained doctors.

Dr Ntabe believes Malawi should "bond" its medical staff, ensuring they serve several years in the local system once they have completed their training. He also wants foreign governments that hire Malawi's medical staff to pay compensation for the cost of training doctors and nurses to replace them.

Estimated critical shortages of doctors, nurses and midwives, by WHO region

WHO region	Number of countries		In countries with shortages		
	Total	With shortages	Total workforce	Estimated shortage	Percentage increase required
Africa	46	36	590 198	817 992	139
Americas	35	5	93 603	37 886	40
South-East Asia	11	6	2 332 054	1 164 001	50
Europe	52	0	NA	NA	NA
Eastern Mediterranean	21	7	312 613	306 031	98
Western Pacific	27	3	27 260	32 560	119
World	192	57	3 355 728	2 358 470	70

NA, not applicable.

World Health Organization
April 06

WHO

The United Nations is the author of the original material.

The brain drain, says Dr Gbary, means the vacancy rate for nurses and doctors in Malawi is so high that even when donors offer funds "it is impossible to use them because the people are simply not there to work."

Some hospitals have resorted to hiring local staff out of retirement in a bid to make up the shortfalls.

But the lure of higher pay in the developed world is not the only reason behind the brain drain. With nearly 15 per cent of Malawi's adult population infected with HIV, many medical staff have themselves become ill with Aids or died.

The Aids epidemic has added to the burden on those who remain, which in turn has encouraged many in Malawi's state health sector to seek higher paid work and better conditions in private and non-governmental organisations—or even in different professions.

"It becomes frustrating working for the state," says Dr Roderick Narikungari, who quit after 10 years to join Medecins sans Frontiéres in Malawi. "There was a lack of resources . . . but I was being moved away from treatment into administration." He says many of his colleagues have left for richer neighbours such as Botswana as well as the UK.

Robin Broadhead, head of the College of Medicine in Blantyre, Malawi, says: "The brain drain is a sheer disgrace. But you can't expect to keep doctors here in artificial slavery."

Desperate government officials are now hunting for scapegoats. In particular, western academic institutions are being accused of luring talent away from treatment to research.

"Our people are rushing (to the institutions) where they are paid a lot more, do a lot less, sitting and filling out research forms," says Dr Ntabe. "It's ridiculous."

Such views now threaten a groundbreaking clinical trial planned by the University of North Carolina to test whether the Aids drug tenofovir can be used as a prophylactic. The trial is supported by the non-government group Family Health International.

Dr Francis Martinson, UNC's programme officer in Malawi, rejects such claims. "The government is always searching to blame everyone apart from itself. Most people have left the system because they don't like it."

He argues that UNC, which employs 70 medical staff in Malawi on salaries up to twice state levels, ensures nearly all spend substantial time on clinical work. It has also helped to fund facilities.

Ironically, while the WHO argues that Africa needs another 1m medical staff to meet basic health goals, it has recruited several of Malawi's top doctors. Others have gone into national politics and government, such as Dr Ntabe himself.

For now, Dr Ntabe and his colleagues see no obvious cure for the brain drain. Africa's efforts to improve healthcare will, it seems, continue to suffer.

Botswana Health Care System Needs Dialogue

By Dr. Vincent Molelekwa
Mmegi/The Reporter, September 1, 2006

In my previous communication (Molelekwa, *Mmegi* 03/08/06), I showed why lack of retention of the local doctor in the public health care sector is indirectly related to the current hospital-based rotational system. I argued that it delays rapid entry into specialist training, retards progression and has a multiplier effect on remuneration issues. Now I would deal with remuneration, workload and unsocial hours. I would further shed light into reasons why newly qualified local doctors delay returning home upon completion of undergraduate training. A sincere rebuttal of Dr Edward Tlholwe Maganu's recent manuscript entitled "Rights without responsibilities", (*Mmegi*, 02/08/06), would also be tabled without prejudice.

Let's revisit the hard facts on the ground. Since the early 90s, government has been able to retain about 50 local doctors in the public funded hospitals. Out of every 10 doctors in the public-funded hospitals, about 9 are expatriates. Extrapolating from Central Statistics Office figures, March 2006, and other peripheral data the current number of doctors in public hospitals is about 540, with about 54 local doctors (the more optimistic figure being 60). Consider that the majority of these expatriates are paid much better than their local counterparts! On average, a local doctor is retained for about 3–5 years in government hospitals before voting with his/her feet for greener pastures. All this while, reasons for the massive exodus of the local expertise to the private sector have been well-articulated. All this time the health ministry has offered the same ineffective solutions.

If you asked the question why we have so many expatriate doctors you would be told because local doctors don't stay in public hospital based medicine. If you asked why they don't stay you would be told because they say they are not paid enough. If you asked why they are not paid enough, it would be answered, because there is no money. But if you asked how can you afford to pay all the about 500 or so expatriate doctors so much money and waste so much in their keeping, you would be considered a moron! Herein lies the naivety in this irrational state of affairs! That it is ok to spend exorbitantly on the expatriate doctor at the cost of retention of local expertise! Doesn't it make sense to pay the local doctor as much as his expatriate colleague, retain him in the public funded hospital, with time reduce reliance on expatriates and eventually localise the important posts?

Solutions to the haemorrhage of local talent have ranged from coercion to self-sacrifice on the basis of patriotism, persuasive arguments that "local doctors deserve to be treated bad because they cost

> The local doctor has never accepted, does not and will not accept his/her current conditions of service.

the nation too much to train" and burying of the heads in the sand by the authorities at the suggestion of reforms. This carry-on continues until the self imposed precarious indifference to the pleas of the local doctor leads to a severe critical shortage of manpower and specialists. Then plan B is activated. A transcontinental recruitment of the disadvantaged expatriate doctors. With it a compulsory repulsive inducement package that lures them to work in "the land already flowing with milk and honey." This scandalous negative feed back cycle keeps on rolling on. The question that must be asked is why a solution has not been found to this day. Secondly, why a healthy frank and constructive dialogue has not been entered into between the health ministry and its local employee doc tors in a bid to finding sustainable solutions. The local doctor has never accepted, does not and will not accept his/her current conditions of service. If persuasion is all that was needed, there would be no need for this current debate. Any further burying of heads in the sand would only yield exactly the same results. Consequently, far-reaching health reforms are critical in resolving the current dilemma. This should lead us into pay, work load and unsocial hours often endured with silence by doctors. It should further inevitably transgress into a subject broached and tempered with careful belligerence by Dr. Edward Tlholwe Maganu. That is, whether doctors like other citizens whose education and training has been government sponsored have the right to collective bargaining. That there is shortage of manpower in our hospitals is public knowledge. That this is exacerbated by the lack of retention of the local expertise is the reason why I am at pains to put forward the doctors' side of the current bottleneck.

The issue of unacceptable levels of workload endured in our hospitals has been raised recently by the junior doctors of Botswana in their recent strike. While every citizen would cry foul if expected to work more than a 40hr week, doctors are asked to consider that they were expensive to train when they complain of the impacts of a more than 70hr week they are regularly expected to endure. While every one would ask for a rightful double pay for hours worked in excess of the 40 hr week, doctors are again informed they were expensive to train, there is no money, we are a middle-income country and therefore would only be given 15percent of their salaries for overtime! None of these reasons seem applicable when considering the rights of other citizen employees. For eons doctors have worked unsocial hours in the form of the inherent night time work on a journey of self sacrifice.

The impact of the combined lack of sleep, fatigue owing to shortage of manpower and lack of appreciation of this unsustainable sacrifice has only been recently understood by the public. For it is now recognised that doctors compared to similar professions have some of the highest divorce rates and a similarly higher substance abuse rate. As is the case, the only people that are expected to pickup the pieces are the families of the affected section of the community. When asking to be remunerated in accord with the level of his skill and the conditions of his service, the local doctor is said to be kicking Batswana in their teeth.

Unfortunately, those of this view have failed dismally to retain the local doctor in public hospital-based medicine. This should not come as a surprise as those who are agitating for sacrifice cannot themselves afford to live by the dose of their prescribed medicine! Dr Edward Tlholwe Maganu is his recent communication, perhaps irked by the mentioning of dry bones on the ongoing debate, has rightly (in my view) come to the defence of the status quo.

The force of his argumentation is almost tangible in his assertion that, "These young professionals are essentially appealing to the people of Botswana to sympathise with and condone their staying or moving overseas on the basis of accusations by themselves of government ineptitude or mismanagement of the health sector, and they overlook the large amounts of money that the government (read people) of Botswana invested in their training."

After accusing doctors' demands for fair play as typical of the unjustifiable culture of entitlement, Dr. Maganu argued that these young professionals are saying to the people of Botswana "pay the P2million or whatever it costs to train me in Europe or America, but expect no service from me unless you satisfy certain conditionalities set by myself, relating to levels of pay and so on, that should guarantee me the standard of life I am used to in the developed country where I studied, as well as the same kind of health system."

They are essentially saying they are entitled to this training at the expense of the country and its people, but the country and its people are not entitled to their service. Dr Maganu's argument as framed seems full proof and beyond reproach, but looked carefully it carries with it certain flaws and assumptions that have over the ages led us exactly where we are today. Before going any further, let the reader understand who Dr Maganu is and how it is possible that he differs considerably with the views of the hospital-based doctors of Botswana.

Dr Maganu himself is a deserter; no different in principle to those who deserted hospital-based medicine to look for private practice locally or migrating abroad! The only difference is that while the majority of such doctors are over the seas, he happens to be over the borders! He happens to have left hospital based medicine for a better package in the health ministry—as a permanent secretary! He is currently writing from Dar es Salaam working for WHO. What the reader needs to know is why he left.

The reason is the same as that advanced by the doctors he is accusing as traitors to the course. His motivation to change his job twice is just as much an act of personal preservation and self-gratification as it is a protest against the conditions of service! There is nothing wrong with what he has done, if only he were to be honest. What we now see is a typical Pharisaic tendency of prescribing an ideal life style while the tutor lives otherwise!

Indeed Dr Maganu and like-minded thinkers have repeatedly erred in their thinking that the reasons why newly qualified doctors fail to return home upon immediate completion of their studies is for reasons of pay, substandard health care conditions or perceived life style in the training country! These unjustifiable odiums that have been cast upon these crops of doctors are deliberate, misleading and framed to incite recriminations from the public upon its sons and daughters. May it be known in official and public fora that newly qualified doctors do not immediately return home for want of undergoing specialist training in the shortest possible time! I repeat is has nothing whatsoever to do with what Dr Maganu and company wants the public to believe.

I have dealt with the impact on progression of the current rotational system, lack of continuing medical education and protected training time on the careers of doctors and their families in my previous posting (Molelekwa, *Mmegi* 03/08/06). To read anything beyond reasons advanced here is desperately mischievous.

Doctors need an average of 4 years to specialise after their initial primary degree (I needed 6 years). The author spent 3 years in UB followed by 6 years of medical training. That makes it 9 years of university. To spend another 3–5 years in Botswana before specialty training is not acceptable. This is one point that local doctors differ sharply with officials, a point that must be addressed with urgency. Consequently, doctors do return home, but do not stay in public hospitals for long! Therefore, the reasons why doctors delay returning home after completion of undergraduate training, and the lack of retention are two completely different issues deserving different solutions.

The attitude demonstrated by my colleague is a continuation of the same line of reasoning that he had while in central government. It has not yielded results and yet he recommends exactly the same solution that he did eons ago! The solution for the current impasse lies beyond the box. Only radical reforms that are agreed to both sides will yield long lasting results. It must be a journey shared with understanding and trust. Any untoward vilification of the local doctor will only strengthen his resolve and push him beyond reach!

The second point raised by Dr Maganu is pertinent to the current stalemate. What is immediately admissible is that it is expensive to train a doctor as everyone by now must be aware. The question at

the heart of this debate is whether it is acceptable, reasonable, justifiable and even-handed to mistreat a doctor at the work place as a
down payment for his expensive training? Further, whether a doctor
as a consequence to his expensive training must be made to lose his
right to demand fair play, better remuneration, improved conditions
of service that are commensurate with his level of skill? Further
more, whether it is unpatriotic for doctors with intimate knowledge
of our limited resource base to ask to be remunerated and treated
exactly the same as fellow citizens of different professions with similar standard of training? It is here argued with contempt, by Dr
Maganu, that the local doctor wants pays and conditions of service
that are exactly the same as that of his/her training country! What
Dr Maganu would like the reader to believe is deceptively dishonest,
especially when he himself deserted the hospital-based environment
for better pay packages! The answers to the above questions are a
resounding NO from the point of view of the disaffected local doctors.

If that was not so, they would have remained, rendering thereby
the ongoing debate obsolete. More to this, no amount of persuasion
has in time past, at present or the foreseeable future been successful
to cushion him/her against the unbearable conditions of service and
therefore discouraged him from leaving. When doctors complain of
basic things such as shortage of basic medicines and infrastructure
they are not asking for anything beyond the means of our middle
income economy. Neither, should they be misconstrued as belittling
our hard working authorities.

Often, shortage of medicines and the like are a symptom of a
poorly managed service delivery that can be corrected by taking into
account of positive and negative points in a constructive critical crit-
icism of delivery mechanisms. Clearly, the massive exodus of the
medical local talent into greener pastures is a culmination of a combination of factors whose cause, effect and potential solutions are
irreducible into an infinitesimal singularity of reasoning.

Negotiated packages of reforms that are critical in breaking down
the pervasive cycle of training and failure of retention of the local
cadres deserve to be explored.

Private Sector, Human Resources and Health Franchising in Africa

By Ndola Prata, Dominic Montagu, and Emma Jefferys
Bulletin of the World Health Organization, April 2005

Introduction

Poverty and health are inextricably interrelated, and the poor are especially vulnerable to further impoverishment if faced with the high costs of illness or the death of a family member (*1,2*). Health inequality has been studied using a number of wellness measures. These include health status, health service spending or financing and health service use. The evidence available from multi-country surveys shows large differences between the rich and the poor (*3*). Public spending on curative health care in Africa does not seem to be reaching most of the poor. On average, government subsidies for curative health care are imperfectly targeted and primarily benefit the wealthy (*2*). Although poverty is closely associated with rural areas, the majority of government health-care facilities in Africa are located in urban areas (*4*). The constraints arising from distance from care providers, combined with the uncertainty of receiving the necessary drugs or treatment from public services, too often leave the poor with only two options: locally available private health care providers, or doing without health-care services altogether.

Even where public facilities do exist, equivalent privately delivered services are often perceived by the users to be of higher quality, irrespective of the empirical evidence that often suggests the opposite (*5*). In developing countries, private-sector delivery of primary health care is usually poorly regulated and prices are usually scaled according to the ability-to-pay of the client (*6–8*). As a result, when the poor seek treatment from private providers they are likely to spend a greater proportion of their income on health care, leading to an increased financial burden. This quandary is a form of market failure: the source of health care is often private, but the private sector is not structured to assure quality or affordability of health care. Strategies to improve access to health-care services and products in developing countries need to take into account the health-seeking behaviour of the various socioeconomic groups so that the poor can be protected and served appropriately. In theory, regulation and enforcement can improve private-sector care, but such measures have a limited track record in areas where government presence is already weak.

The limited human resources available to governments necessitate a strategy of greater involvement with the private sector. An increase in government services, when and if it comes, will not be sufficient to increase diagnosis and entry into treatment to reach the rates set by the Millennium Development Goals (*9–11*). The opportunities to intervene with private providers to improve access and quality, ensure equity of prices, and empower clients have been studied both in theory and in practice.

Health franchising is an application of commercial franchising systems to socially motivated health programmes (*12,13*). Individual franchisees operate for-profit outlets or clinics, in accordance with clear and strictly defined clinical and quality guidelines set out in a contractual relationship with the franchiser. As a method of organizing an unstructured private sector, franchising is attractive because it incorporates into one system all of the interventions that have been shown to have some effect individually (training, oversight, performance-based incentives, accreditation and certification, vouchers or other external payment schemes, ongoing support relationships and monitoring). Often called social franchising programmes, these programmes have been used successfully for nearly 10 years by family planning clinics in Asia and Africa, and for essential drug provision and programmes for voluntary counselling and testing for human immunodeficiency virus (HIV) in Africa.

The purpose of the present study was to examine the scale of the private health sector in Africa, its importance for mobilization towards meeting public health goals, and the potential of health franchising to function as a primary mechanism for this mobilization. This was done by determining which strata of society benefit from publicly or privately provided services; by shedding light on the size and composition of health-care providers in sub-Saharan Africa; and by providing evidence that health franchising in Africa has the potential to improve service availability to the poor through large-scale programmes.

Data and Methods

Data on health-care service utilization by socioeconomic status for 22 countries in sub-Saharan Africa were published in the Health Nutrition and Population Poverty Thematic Reports of The World Bank (*3*). Health service use for the treatment of two very common childhood diseases, diarrhoea and acute respiratory infection (ARI), was examined. Treatments for these two diseases can be considered to be good proxies for public services that are either free-of-charge or highly subsidized. For each disease, service use was assessed by socioeconomic status and type of provider (i.e. public or private) for both rural and urban populations. Gwatkin et al. defined socioeconomic status in terms of asset wealth quintiles, gathered through the Demographic and Health Surveys (DHS) household questionnaire (*14*). Provider type was categorized as either public or private. Public facilities included government hospitals, health centres and dispensaries. Private providers included private physicians, mission hospitals and clinics, other private hospitals and clinics, and pharmacies.

Data from an Institute for Health Sector Development (IHSD) study were used to estimate the density of private health-care providers in urban and rural areas. The IHSD study was conducted by local experts, using secondary-source analysis and direct interviews with policy-makers and data managers at the ministerial level in Burkina Faso, Cameroon, Ethiopia, Malawi, Mozambique, Nigeria, Rwanda, Uganda and the United Republic of Tanzania. Further details on the methodology have been published elsewhere (*15*).

The experience of health franchising in Africa is limited and few survey data are available, but a number of established programmes in Asia have conducted studies and produced public and internal data. Data from public and grey-literature sources were collected through referrals obtained during interviews with public health researchers, health franchise managers and donors supporting franchise programmes. Documents were verified and supported by face-to-face interviews with health practitioners and programmes managers directly involved in the direction of all health franchises reviewed for the present study.

Results

Service Utilization by Type of Provider

Table 1 shows the distribution of children aged under 5 years who were ill, and the use of health services for treatment of diarrhoeal disease and ARI, by socioeconomic status, in 22 sub-Saharan African countries. Children from the poorest quintile were more likely to have had a recent illness than the children from the richest quintile. In the 22 countries studied, the poorest families were least likely to seek medical care when a child was ill. The poorest children were also those most likely to live in areas that were underserved by public health-care providers.

In the majority of the sub-Saharan African countries for which DHS data were available, of those children seen by a medical practitioner, the use of public services by the rich was not significantly different from that by the poor. On average, of those children seen by a medical practitioner, most of those from the poorest quintile sought care from private providers for both diarrhoeal disease and ARI (Table 1). The DHS surveys from which these data were taken were nationally representative samples. The reported source of care (i.e. public or private) was therefore inferred from the results to reflect the combined effects of availability of services and choice of provider. The use of private services did not differ significantly between socioeconomic groups, the differences were mainly between those receiving and those not receiving services, with a higher proportion of the poor not receiving any medical services.

In only three of the countries (Namibia, the United Republic of Tanzania and Zambia), did half or more than half of the poorest children receive treatment for ARI from the public health care sector. To further explore the role of the private sector in service provision to poor people, we took the country examples, Mozambique and Uganda, and chose Namibia as being representative of the three outliers.

In Mozambique, of those children who were ill with diarrhoea, the percentage seen at private sector health-care facilities did not differ significantly between socioeconomic groups. Among the children who were ill, even in rural areas, the difference between use of private services by the poor (18.8%) and the rich (21.9%) was not statistically significant (P-value = 0.782). The largest differences seen between rich and poor were in whether or not they received any treatment at all; the richest were most likely to receive care. Mozambique is an example of a country in which the rich made more use of the public services than the poor (45.8% versus 6.4%; P-value < 0.0001 for rural populations).

The use of services for the treatment of acute respiratory diseases in Uganda, exemplifies another group of countries where most of those who sought medical care at any socioeconomic level did so through the private sector. Moreover, of those who were ill, the difference in use of private services between the rural poor (37.9%) and the rural rich (48%) was not statistically significant (P-value = 0.063). In Uganda, the public sector facilities for treating children with respiratory infections were used by only a small fraction across all socioeconomic groups. Nevertheless, even the rural poor made significantly less use (P-value < 0.0001) of the public services (10.6%) than the rich (23.8%).

In Namibia (the outlier) the majority of those seeking medical treatment for diarrhoeal disease did so through the public sector. Even in rural areas, the comparison of private facility use across socioeconomic groups was not statistically significant (P-values >

Table 1. **Mean percentages of ill children and reported use of health services for treatment of diarrhoeal disease and acute respiratory infections by socioeconomic group from selected African countries**[a] (population 0–5 years old ill 2 weeks preceding the survey)

	% ill					% those ill who were seen by a medical practitioner					% of those seen by a medical practitioner who were seen in public facilities				
	Poor-est	2nd quintile	Mid	4th quintile	Rich-est	Poor-est	2nd quintile	Mid	4th quintile	Rich-est	Poor-est	2nd quintile	Mid	4th quintile	Rich-est
Diarrhoeal disease	24.5	23.3	22.5	22.6	18.2	34.3	36.2	37.5	40.8	47.3	22.7	23.7	25.2	28.5	30.4
Acute respiratory infections	17.9	17.8	16.0	15.5	14.3	33.2	38.9	43.9	46.7	59.1	26.2	30.3	34.8	37.5	42.5

[a] Benin, Burkina Faso, Cameroon, Central African Republic, Chad, Comorros, Côte d'Ivoire, Ghana, Kenya, Madagascar, Malawi, Mali, Mozambique, Namibia, Niger, Nigeria, Senegal, United Republic of Tanzania, Togo, Uganda, Zambia, Zimbabwe.
Source: Data compiled from individual country reports by Gwatkin et al. (2000). Socio-Economic Differences in Health, Nutrition, and Population Health Nutrition and Population Poverty Thematic Group of The World Bank.

0.05). However, the use of private sector health-care for childhood diseases, although much lower than the public sector use, did not differ significantly between socioeconomic groups (comparison of proportions public versus private with P-values > 0.05). The private sector reached poor and rich equally.

Distribution of Private Sector Health-care in Sub-Saharan Africa

According to a recent IHSD study on private sector health care in sub-Saharan Africa (15), the size of the independent private sector in sub-Saharan Africa varied enormously between countries. On average, doctors and pharmacists were the most likely to operate privately, and they were mostly concentrated in urban centres. The largest numbers of nurses operating privately were in Cameroon, Malawi, Nigeria, Uganda and the United Republic of Tanzania (12%, 10%, 25%, 8% and 13%, respectively, of the nurses operating in each country). In all of the countries included in the study, some

---

Governments in sub-Saharan Africa increasingly regard public-private partnerships as a necessary step towards expanding access to basic health care services.

---

staff employed by the public sector also worked in the private sector, although the estimated proportion varied between countries. Some of the countries had no specific laws or regulations either authorizing or prohibiting the practice of working in both the public and private sectors (Ethiopia, Malawi, Mozambique and Nigeria), although in many countries such a practice was informally recognized, as long as it occurred outside the working hours of the main employment.

Health Franchising

Our study demonstrated that large numbers of the poor received care from private providers. Governments in sub-Saharan Africa increasingly regard public-private partnerships as a necessary step towards expanding access to basic health-care services (16,17). As a result, there is a need for systems that can organize existing private providers to ensure the availability of diagnostics and treatment for public health priority illnesses. The components of availability must include provider competence, diagnostic capacity, existing and assured supply of treatment medications, and pricing or payment exemptions that ensure the affordability of these services.

A number of schemes involving private providers have had an effect on some of these components. Voucher systems have increased the affordability of specific health-care treatments, but are prohibitively expensive to manage through large numbers of service-delivery points (*18,19*). Postgraduate education for private providers has led to improvements in the quality of clinical care, but the benefits declined over time in the absence of systems for continued regular engagement with public and private systems (*20–22*). Regulation can be effective, but has a poor track record of continued enforcement in Africa (*6,7*). Accreditation and certification systems have worked well for hospitals in wealthy and middle-income countries, but have had little success in poor developing countries (*23*). There are no accreditation and certification programmes that have had proven impacts on private solo practitioners. Public-private partnerships, where governments take the initiative to contact and encourage referrals from private health-care providers such as pulmonary specialists, sometimes including supply to the private provider of free treatment medication, have demonstrated successes for tuberculosis control, but no studies on integration with other diseases have yet been documented (*24*).

Health franchising is an attractive innovation for integrating private providers into public health programmes because it combines critical aspects of all of the initiatives above. Health franchising is based on contractual agreements with medical providers, in which the providers sell services (often subsidized so that there is a lower cost to the end-user) and receive member-specific benefits. Such benefits include the right to use the franchise brand; training; access to certain drugs; business loans; prestige from name-association; and advertising. Thanks to these benefits, the experience has been that franchisees usually enjoy a profitable business and increased clientele, and that client satisfaction is higher in users of franchised clinics than in those who use equivalent non-franchised clinics (*25*).

Client satisfaction is a result of the contract: for the franchisee, membership benefits are conditional upon the delivery of quality care. Quality regulations—for example, on clinic cleanliness, patient interaction, and application of appropriate clinical protocols—are monitored by the franchiser through client exit interviews, tracking of drug sales, and in some cases trained actors may pose as clients ("mystery clients"). If the franchisee fails to follow the regulations set out in the initial contract, the franchise is revoked. As long as the value of the opportunity is greater than the value of breaking the rules and there is a credible threat of enforcement, franchisees follow the rules and self-regulate, lowering the overall cost of monitoring. This self-regulation makes this particular system of service expansion and quality improvement cost-effective in a way that is only possible because the goals of the provider (selling medicine and treating patients) are aligned with the goals of the franchiser (ensuring availability and appropriate care).

The specific model of franchising adopted varies depending on how critical it is to maintain quality assurance and compliance of providers with standards. Unlike other systems for involving private providers in the pursuit of public health goals, franchising can promise and deliver a high quality of care and it has been proven to work on a large scale. The experiences of the Greenstar programmes in Pakistan, Janani in India, Child and Family Welfare shops in Kenya, and many others have demonstrated the potential for a franchise model to greatly increase service availability through the mobilization of existing private health care human resources.

One attraction of health franchising is that it has been successful in vastly different societies. In India, a health franchise has improved the sexual health of inter-city truck drivers through provision of education, contraceptives and diagnosis and treatment of sexually transmitted infections near motorway rest stops (*13*). In Nicaragua, Marie Stopes International, a British non-profit organization specializing in reproductive health, runs a similar health franchise for sexual health services. The Well-Family Midwife Clinic franchise in the Philippines provides midwives trained in safe birth practices to attend deliveries through more than 100 outlets.

> One attraction of health franchising is that it has been successful in vastly different societies.

The franchise system has also proven successful in sub-Saharan Africa: in Ethiopia the Biruh Tesfa (Ray of Hope) programmes increased contraceptive use by 30% among the 10 million people covered by its 92 clinics (*25*). In Zimbabwe, New Start franchised testing and counselling for HIV; this had increased monthly visits from 230 in 1999 to 4000 in 2003 (*26*). In Kenya, the Sustainable Healthcare Enterprise Foundation's Child and Family Welfare Shops (SHEF/CFW) programmes have provided affordable generic drugs through franchised community health workers. SHEF/CFW generates income from 80% of its franchisees, despite serving low-income customers in rural areas (*27*). Survey data from India, Nepal, Pakistan and elsewhere have shown that clients respond positively to franchise brands, and that the volume of branded services (offered by a provider and quality-assured through oversight by the agency) provided by franchisees is higher than that provided by equivalent non-franchised private providers. It is difficult to make quality measures in the private sector, but one unpublished study from Nepal (D Montague, personal communication) found that counselling provided to mystery clients was more complete and more objective when provided by franchise members than when provided by non-franchise members. A multi-country survey of franchises found that patient-to-staff ratios were significantly lower at franchised facilities than at non-franchised facilities across a number of franchise programmes in Africa and Asia (*28*). The existing evidence remains limited, but indicates that franchising of private providers improves both accessibility and quality of services.

Discussion

Evidence from DHS data confirm earlier studies that have shown that public sector services disproportionately serve the wealthy in developing countries (*2*). Our analysis has further clarified the role of the private sector in filling the gap left by the absence of public sector facilities in serving the poor. The use of private health care for the treatment of childhood diseases does not differ significantly by socioeconomic group. In most countries the poor must usually choose between using private services and not using any health services at all.

A recent review of interventions focusing on improving the quality of health care provided for children by the private sector concluded that the experience with the private sector offered considerable promise for improving child health (*29*). The importance of private providers is especially great today in light of the current challenges of acquired immunodeficiency syndrome (AIDS) and tuberculosis. In

---

It is critical for African governments to actively engage existing private health-care providers in rapidly expanding the availability of health-care services to low-income populations.

Africa, many poor people seek care for tuberculosis and sexually transmitted diseases from private providers because of the stigma these diseases carry (*30,31*).

Extrapolating from the context of need and the health delivery systems currently operating in Africa, our study has concluded that it is critical for African governments to actively engage existing private health-care providers in rapidly expanding the availability of health-care services to low-income populations. Despite the challenges in Africa, the experience of programmes around the world leads us to believe that a system to group and improve the quality of existing private providers would be both viable and beneficial to the poor in a number of countries. Franchising provides an attractive addition to the available tools for leveraging existing human resources and offers a system for standardizing the outputs from a heterogeneous group of practitioners. In addition, it can potentially increase human resources: it works with existing private practitioners who are currently outside public health programming and are almost certainly not providing quality priority disease care for the poor due to restricted drug supplies or lack of ability and support. The inclusion of these providers in public health campaigns is likely to result in a net gain for national programmes.

As the governments in Africa are increasingly challenged by the demands of treating AIDS, and pressure from The World Bank and other donors to expand the reach of public-private partnerships, there is a need for new ideas to involve the hitherto unutilized human resources available in the private sector. There are few models that can be adopted to effectively motivate private providers to support public health goals. Health franchising has a track record of successes and provides a possible solution to this urgent and challenging problem.

References

1. The World Bank. *World Development Report 1990: Poverty.* Washington, DC: World Bank/Oxford University Press; 1990.

2. Castro-Leal F, Dayton J, Demery L, Mehra K. Public spending on health care in Africa: do the poor benefit? *Bulletin of the World Health Organization* 2000;78:66–74.

3. Gwatkin DR. Health inequalities and the health of the poor: what do we know? What can we do? *Bulletin of the World Health Organization* 2000;78:3–18.

4. Hjortsberg CA, Mwikisa CN. Cost of access to health services in Zambia. *Health Policy and Planning* 2002;17:71–7.

5. Brugha R, Zwi A. Improving the quality of private sector delivery of public health services: challenges and strategies. *Health Policy and Planning* 1998;13:107–20.

6. Hongoro C, Kumaranayake L. Do they work? Regulating for-profit providers in Zimbabwe. *Health Policy and Planning* 2000;15:368–77.

7. Kumaranayake L, Mujinja P, Hongoro C, Mpembeni R. How do countries regulate the health sector? Evidence from Tanzania and Zimbabwe. *Health Policy and Planning* 2000;15:357–67.

8. Soderlund N, Tangcharoensathien V. Health sector regulation— understanding the range of responses from Government. *Health Policy and Planning* 2000;15:347–8.

9. Leonard D. *Africa's changing markets for health and veterinary services.* New York: Saint Martin's Press; 2000.

10. Ngalande-Banda E, Walt G. The private health sector in Malawi: opening Pandora's box? *Journal of International Development* 1995;7:403–22.

11. Rosen J, Conly S. *Getting down to business.* Washington, DC: Population Action International; 1999.

12. Montagu D. Franchising of health services in low-income countries. *Health Policy and Planning.* 2002;17:121–30.

13. Smith E. *Social franchising reproductive health services: can it work?* London: Marie Stopes International; 2002. Report No. 5.

14. Gwatkin DR, Rustein S, Johnson K, Pande R, Wagstaff A. *Socioeconomic differences in health, nutrition, and population.* Washington, DC: World Bank; 2000.

15. Jefferys E. *Evaluating the private sector potential for franchising TB and HIV/AIDS diagnosis and care in Sub-Saharan Africa.*

London: Institute for Health Sector Development; 2004. Available from:
URL: http://www.ihsd.org/docs/JefferysFranchising04.pdf

16. Lambo E, Sambo LG. Health sector reform in sub-Saharan Africa: a synthesis of country experiences. *East African Medical Journal* 2003;80 (6 Suppl):S1–20.

17. Sekwat A. Health financing reform in sub-Saharan Africa: major constraints, goals, and strategies. *Journal of Health Care Finance* 2003;29:67–78.

18. Mushi AK, Schellenberg JR, Mponda H, Lengeler C. Targeted subsidy for malaria control with treated nets using a discount voucher system in Tanzania. *Health Policy Planning* 2003;18:163–71.

19. Gorter A, Sandiford P, Rojas Z, Salvetto M. *Competitive voucher schemes for health, background paper*. Washington, DC: Central American Health Institute/World Bank; 2003.

20. Ibrahim S, Isani Z. Evaluation of doctors trained at Diarrhoea Training Unit of National Institute of Child Health, Karachi. *Journal of the Pakistan Medical Association* 1997;47:7–11.

21. Choudhry AJ, Mubasher M. Factors influencing the prescribing patterns in acute watery diarrhoea. *Journal of the Pakistan Medical Association* 1997;47:32–5.

22. Luby S, Zaidi N, Rehman S, Northrup R. Improving private practitioner sick-child case management in two urban communities in Pakistan. *Tropical Medicine and International Health.* 2002;7:210–9.

23. Shawn C. External assessment of health care. *BMJ* 2001;322:851–4.

24. Lonnroth K, Uplekar M, Arora VK, Juvekar S, Lan NT, Mwaniki D, et al. Public-private mix for DOTS implementation: what makes it work? *Bulletin of the World Health Organization* 2004;82:580–6.

25. Stephenson R, Tsui AO, Sulzbach S, Bardsley P, Bekele G, Giday T, et al. Franchising reproductive health services. *Health Services Research* 2004;39:2053–80.

26. Population Services International. *New Hope with New Start. Vol. 2004*. Washington, DC: Population Services International; 2004.

27. Sustainable Healthcare Enterprise Foundation. *Facts about CFW Vol. 2004*. Minneapolis, U.S.A: Sustainable Healthcare Enterprise Foundation; 2004.

28. Sulzbach S. *Franchising reproductive health services*. Minneapolis: Population Association of America; 2002.

29. Waters H, Hatt L, Peters D. Working with the private sector for child health. *Health Policy and Planning* 2003;18:127–37.

30. Berman P. Organization of ambulatory care provision: a critical determinant of health system performance in developing countries. *Bulletin of the World Health Organization* 2000;78:791–802.
31. Brugha R. Antiretroviral treatment in developing countries: the peril of neglecting private providers. *BMJ* 2003;326:1382–4.

Defining Minimum Standards of Practice for Incorporating African Traditional Medicine into HIV/AIDS Prevention, Care, and Support

A Regional Initiative in Eastern and Southern Africa

By Jaco Homsy, M.D., M.P.H., et al.
The Journal of Alternative and Complementary Medicine, 2004

Introduction

African Traditional Medicine is characterized by a holistic approach to the spirit–mind–body concept of health, embracing people, animals, plants, and inanimate objects in an inseparable whole from which all beings derive their living and healing forces. In many resource-poor settings of Africa, a majority of people living with HIV/AIDS continue to depend on and choose traditional healers and herbal treatments for psychosocial counseling and health care (UNAIDS, 2002). This is not only because healers and herbs are more available and accessible to their communities than biomedical doctors or drugs, but also because the majority of Africans believe in the usefulness and power of traditional medicine. However, many conventional health workers distrust traditional medicine (TM) and THs, while healers have little information about AIDS and lack standardized training and practices. In addition, herbal treatments have often never been rigorously evaluated, are not always properly prepared or standardized, and are frequently poorly packaged and preserved, limiting their usefulness and accessibility to the immediate production site (Burford et al, 2000; Rukangira, 2001).

The idea of the Regional Initiative on Traditional Medicine and AIDS in Eastern & Southern Africa was spearheaded by the Ugandan nongovernmental organization Traditional and Modern Health Practitioners Together Against AIDS and Other Diseases, in Kampala, (www.thetauganda.org) in 2001 Traditional and Modern Health Practitioners Together Against AIDS and Other Diseases (THETA), Kampala, Uganda. to promote a concerted, systematic, and sustained effort at both local and regional levels to support and validate African Traditional Medicine on several fronts in relation to HIV/ AIDS (Homsy et al, 2003). A regional consultation that took tice around six predefined themes regarding the involvement of traditional healers and traditional medicine in HIV/ AIDS prevention, care, and treatment. These standards, summarized below, along with related implementation strategies, represent the first regional and participatory attempt to enhance the validity and credibility of African traditional medicine while preserving its identity and diversity.

Proposed Standards

1. *Evaluation of traditional medicine*—One of the main limitations in the use of traditional medicines is the lack of scientific evidence regarding their effectiveness (Rukangira, 2001). The following recommendations were made in accordance with the World Health Organization (WHO) guidelines (WHO, 2001) and, in addition to the WHO guidelines, a number of practical incremental steps were proposed, defining feasible field-adapted protocols able to gather rapid and sufficient evidence to validate traditional medicine:

   - Evaluation of traditional medicine should be preceded and guided by information-gathering on purported efficacy and safety (document review, literature search, interviews and discussions with patients and healers, and ethnomedical evidence)

   - Observational studies should be conducted to generate further information on safety and assess preliminary indicative efficacy. Minimum methods were outlined for enrolment and follow-up of participants, care for side-effects and referral, administration of the traditional treatment, and conduct of the study.

   - Standard clinical trial methodology was deemed inappropriate and too costly for evaluating the numerous preparations already in use by millions of people including persons living with HIV/AIDS (PLHAs) throughout Africa. New practical and acceptable research tools need to be developed in accordance with the minimum regulatory requirements that WHO has developed, for registration and use of traditional medicines in Africa with respect to quality, safety, and efficacy (World Health Organization, 2001, and in press).

   - Results should be shared with the primary beneficiaries of the studies (PLHAs and traditional healers) as well as disseminated to the community and other stakeholders, through both verbal communications and document dissemination.

   - Accessibility to the traditional treatment tested should be ensured through the use of local ingredients and through their processing and packaging in a low-cost form suitable for ease of administration and distribution.

2. *Spiritual healing*—Spiritual healing was defined as entirely distinct from witchcraft. It was described as a process mediated through spiritual or divine powers not associated with use of medicine or physical body manipulation, unless so directed/instructed by spirits. Different levels of spiritual specialization were described, including a hierarchy among spirits, ranging from junior to senior spirits. Characteristics of the practice of spiritual healing were outlined. The practice should:

- Be accepted by the community

- Have no negative social or physical connotations

- Be provided free of charge; community/clients only make voluntary contributions.

In addition:

- The time of service should be a spiritual choice and the service should include guidance, counseling, healing, review of cultural practices, peace promotion, security (protection from malevolent spirits), and advocacy for good practices. Services can address past, present, and future issues, and should never involve sacrifices.

- Personal attributes of the spiritual medium/healer were defined as persons or animals chosen/sent by spirits (hence, not always from the community), who often do not stay in the same place and never choose who they are, how they work, and where they work from. Spiritual healing usually involves team work with associates and assistants.

- Ethical standards of practice include the observance of confidentiality, the option for clients to make appointments, and the dependence of the healer on her/his guiding spirits.

- The healer's workplace can be any place recognized by the spirit, but the place should be recognized and respected by the community and be freely accessible to all members without fear.

- Spiritual healers may use various implements, including spears, walking sticks, pipes for smoking, tobacco, traditional cloth, animal skins, calabashes, and fireplaces.

3. *Prevention and care*—TH have been shown to be effective HIV/AIDS educators, counselors, and sources of referrals (Green, 1995, King and Homsy, 1997, UNAIDS, 2002). Communities, traditional healer clients and practitioners, (including, traditional healers and biomedical health practitioners), should be

trained/empowered in the following minimum aspects of HIV prevention and care:

- Cultural beliefs and practices
- Basic and updated information on prevention and care for sexually transmitted diseases (STDs), HIV/AIDS, and tuberculosis (TB)
- Infection control
- Identification of danger signs to enable THs to make referrals
- Integration of biomedical and traditional counseling approaches on STDs, HIV/AIDS, and TB, including client counseling, support, and referral

In addition:

- Training methods should be adapted to TH characteristics: participatory techniques, experience sharing, case studies, role plays have proven to be most adequate.

Training should be an opportunity to share information and knowledge in a mutually respectful way between traditional healing practitioners and biomedical health practitioners, thereby building understanding and trust between the two groups of practitioners, enabling easy referral. At a minimum, traditional healers should be able to give clinically accurate information on STDs, HIV/AIDS, and TB to their clients and community members, identify signs and symptoms of clinical emergencies, refer patients to appropriate health facilities, and demonstrate skills in counseling and information sharing (King and Homsy, 1997; World Health Organization, 2004b).

Referrals should be emphasized both ways (from traditional healing practitioners to biomedical health practitioners and vice versa) and referral systems (including forms) should be introduced in program areas. Biomedical workers should be encouraged to refer patients whose conditions do not respond to biomedical treatments or for which treatments are unavailable or inaccessible, such as chronic skin conditions, mental illness, epilepsy, and spiritual problems. Finally, biomedical health practitioners should demonstrate positive attitudes towards traditional healers/traditional medicine.

4. *Standardisation, processing, and packaging of herbal medicine*—Another important limitation to the use of traditional medicine is the lack of standardized methods and technology regarding the processing, packaging, and labeling of traditional medicine. Minimum recommendations for collecting, processing, and storage of traditional medicines include:

- Proper selection and botanical identification of raw material

- Documented harvesting including location, geographical area, month, date, and time
- Controlled conditioning for temperature, moisture content, light exposure, and drying method
- Controlled storage conditions including good ventilation, protection from light/UV rays (dark room), adequate temperature, and wooden racks.

In addition:

- Accurate selection and identification of correct plants for particular usage should be guided by traditional healers taking into account season, time, and geographical region.
- Minimum extraction standards should ensure hygiene of mechanical extraction devices and using appropriate methods for volatile products and nonvolatile products.
- Storage of extracts/processed medicine should preferably make use of properly covered glass containers. Traditional healers should be encouraged to prepare small quantities (2 days' worth) and store them in a cool place away from direct sunlight.

Minimum standards for the packaging and labeling of traditional medicine preparations of individual traditional healers were differentiated from commercial preparations. Traditional healers should use pots and wooden containers, should not store liquid preparations for more than 2 days in bamboo containers, and should label products with the names of herbs and other ingredients, the dates of collection and packaging, indications and dosages recommended, and methods of application and storage.

Commercial preparations should avoid the use of polythenes and use airtight containers and sterile glass containers for suspensions, solutions, and injectables. Labeling should include the botanical/scientific names and quantities of each ingredient; the date of manufacture and expiration; appropriate dosages for adults, children, and infants; and any known contraindications and other warnings, as appropriate. These standards should be in keeping with the WHO Guidelines on Registration of Traditional Medicines in the WHO African Region (Kasilo et al., in press).

5. *Indigenous knowledge*—African indigenous knowledge on health should be understood as embracing the whole body of knowledge, rites, and practices in the artistic, technological, and medical realms that are unique to the cultures and people of Africa (Naur, 2001). African indigenous knowledge on health should be related to the spiritual, herbal, and technical knowledge, rites, and practices that have been developed and used for generations to heal and alleviate all sorts of physical, emotional, and spiritual ailments in Africa.

Indigenous knowledge on health comprises a number of specializations including, but not limited to:

- Herbal medicine, including the use of animal and mineral products

- Traditional counseling

- Bone setting/surgical procedures

- Preventive traditional medicine

- Spiritual healing

- Traditional midwifery

- Nutritional advice.

Herbal medicine may be used in combination with any of the other practices.

The protection of herbal medicine as indigenous knowledge on health should imply the development of sustainable and traditionally acceptable practices for the cultivation, harvesting, processing, utilization, dissemination, and conservation of medicinal plants (Etkin, 1998). In addition, the protection of the various practices that constitute indigenous knowledge on health should require that each specialty be documented, analyzed, evaluated, validated, and attributed in terms of ownership.

6. *Intellectual property rights*—Protection of intellectual property rights requires information on community needs, incremental documentation at various levels, and the design of model agreements to support collaborative research involving biomedical and traditional health practitioners. Although the minimum standards for legal protection of intellectual property rights will vary depending on specific national contexts (Timmermans, 2003), the following universal practices/approaches were recommended:

- Sensitize communities, THs, and groups involved in collaboration with traditional healers and the traditional medicine sector about intellectual property rights related to IKH and TM

- Give priority to national/local heritage (e.g., protection of traditional sites/areas)

- Use available legal instruments to protect sources (including providers/traditional healers), processes, and products

- Use the Organization for African Unity (OAU) Model Law to advocate for adoption of appropriate national/local legislation to protect IKH (OAU, 1998)

- Comply with recently developed WHO "Policy and Legislative Guidelines on Intellectual Property Rights for Indigenous and

Traditional Medicine in WHO African Region" as a template for adaptation by countries (World Health Organization, 2004a)

- Devise innovative mechanisms for settling complex issues involving key players, such as the establishment of community trusts for indigenous knowledge on health ownership, benefit sharing, and other ways to distribute the proceeds that may arise from the development of useful traditional remedies

In any case,

- Communities or individuals should not sell intellectual property rights, but license them under legal agreements (Fourmile. 1999)
- Public and community health and wealth should prevail over individual and corporate interests (World Trade Organization, 2001).

Implementation Strategies and the Way Forward

Six main strategies were identified to chart the way forward:

1. Promote and implement regional and local multidisciplinary collaborative projects involving modern and traditional health practitioners using the proposed standards within international guidelines established by WHO, UNAIDS, and other recognized bodies. These may include research projects, the establishment of dual clinics (offering modern diagnostics and traditional and modern care), herbal medicinal gardens and nurseries, all of which should intensify partnerships with relevant players at local, national, and regional levels (e.g., healers' and/or growers' associations for conservation of medicinal plants; clergy or politicians to de-stigmatize African TM; health professionals for research).
2. Strengthen networking, information, and dissemination on African TM among regional partners to:
   - Document and learn from best-practice examples
   - Organize regional training programs and exchange visits
   - Build traditional healers' capacity to document their knowledge, experiences, and successes
   - Set up a regional database(s) on various traditional medicine capacities in the region, accessible from the Worldwide Web.

These strategies should be supported further by the upcoming WHO document on Tools for Documenting African Traditional Medicine (World Health Organization, 2003)

3. Reaffirm the primary status of African Traditional Medicine and African indigenous knowledge in African health systems by advocating for:

   - A legal framework that supports the independence and identity of African Traditional Medicine and for which standards should not be solely Western-based

   - Increased public and private investment in TM

   - The addition of African TM to national health services and to formal medical curriculum and training

   - Access to information on indigenous knowledge on health and the regulation of its exploitation.

4. Support traditional medicine institutional development at local, national, and regional levels via:

   - Active contribution to the formulation/revision of national traditional medicine legislation and interim legal tools to strengthen, legalize, and regulate the training requirements, codes, and standards of practice of African Traditional Medicine and related intellectual property and indigenous knowledge using WHO generic tools for institutionalization of traditional medicine as models for adaptation

   - Establishing representative traditional medicine bodies such as a national traditional medicine commission to speak for the profession or body of interested lawyers to represent traditional healers' interests

   - Fostering debates balancing individual, corporate, and community interests related to intellectual property issues

   - Building regional alliances to promote/advocate for traditional medicine.

5. Plan and implement sensitization and education campaigns at local, national, and regional levels aiming particularly at biomedical health practitioners, schools, teacher training colleges, the media, the clergy, parliamentarians, and other relevant bodies of government.

6. Promote the Regional Initiative on Traditional Medicine and AIDS via information dissemination among traditional healers, traditional healers associations and their leaders, supporting regional collaborative programs, defining a strategy to enhance national representation/inclusiveness, raise funds, and implement the way forward for all partners, and select and develop regional Centers of Excellence on traditional medicine in specific areas of practice.

Conclusions

The seeds of the Regional Initiative on Traditional Medicine and HIV/AIDS in Eastern and Southern Africa have been planted. The next challenge is to nurture and bring them into fruition, just like a precious medicinal plant with properties we are only starting to rediscover.

Acknowledgments

We would like to thank Professor Charles Wambebe of the WHO Regional Office for Africa for his helpful comments and suggestions in reviewing this paper.

References

Burford G, Bodeker G, Kabatesi D, Gemmill B, Rukangira E. Traditional medicine and HIV/AIDS in Africa: A report from the International Conference on Medicinal Plants, Traditional Medicine and Local Communities in Africa (a parallel session to the Fifth Conference of the Parties to the Convention on Biological Diversity, Nairobi, Kenya, May 16–19, 2000). J Altern Complement Med 2000;6:457–471.

Etkin NL. Indigenous patterns of conserving biodiversity: Pharmacologic implications. J Ethnopharmacol 1998;63:233–245.

Fourmile H. International issues related to intellectual ownership, the biota and indigenous peoples. Symposium on Scholarship, Intellectual Ownership and the Law, National Academies Forum, National Library of Australia, Canberra, Australia, July 15–16, 1999. Online document at: www.naf.org.au/summary.htm#Fourmile. Accessed October 18, 2004.

Green E. The participation of African traditional healers in AIDS/STD prevention programs. AIDS Link 1995;36:14–15.

Homsy J, King R, Tenywa J. Building a regional initiative for traditional medicine and AIDS in eastern and southern Africa. African Health Monitor 2003;4:24–26.

Kasilo, MJ, Soumbey-Alley, E, Wambebe, C and Chatora, R. Overview of the situation of traditional medicine in the WHO African region. In: Global Atlas on Traditional and Complimentary Medicine—Perspectives on Policy and Practice. World Health Organization Kobe Centre, Japan, 2004:in press.

King R, Homsy J. Involving traditional healers in AIDS education and counselling in sub-saharan Africa: A review. AIDS 97: A Year in Review 1997:S217–S225.

Naur M. Indigenous knowledge and HIV/AIDS: Ghana and Zambia. Online document at: www.worldbank.org/afr/ik/iknt30.pdf Accessed September 17, 2004.

Organisation of African Unity. The Model Law of the Organisation of African Unity on Community Rights and on the Control of Access to Biological Resources. 1998 Online document at: www.grain.org/docs/ouamodellaw-2000-en.pdf. Accessed September 17, 2004.

Rukangira E. Medicinal Plants and Traditional Medicine in Africa: Constraints and Challenges. Sustainable Development International; 4:179–184. Online document at: www.sustdev.org/journals/edition.04/download/ed4.pdfs/sdi4_179.pdf. Accessed September 17, 2004.

Timmermans K. Intellectual property rights and traditional medicine: Policy dilemmas at the interface. Soc Sci Med 2003;57(4): 745–756.

UNAIDS. Ancient Remedies, New Disease: Increasing Access to AIDS Prevention and Care in collaboration with traditional healers. Geneva: UNAIDS Best Practices Collection, 2002.

World Health Organization. WHO/AFRO Protocol for the Evaluation of Herbal Preparations Used for the Treatment of HIV/AIDS. Brazzaville, Congo: WHO Regional Office for Africa, 2001.

World Health Organization. Tools for Institutionalising Traditional Medicine in National Health Systems in the WHO African Region. Brazzaville, Congo: WHO Regional Office for Africa, 2003.

World Health Organization. Policy and Legislative Guidelines on Intellectual Property Rights for Indigenous Knowledge and Traditional Medicine in WHO African Region. Brazzaville, Congo: WHO Regional Office for Africa, 2004a.

World Health Organization. Guidelines for Registration of Traditional Medicines in the WHO African Region. WHO Regional Office for Africa, Brazzaville, Congo. In press.

World Health Organization. Chronic HIV Care with ARV Therapy-Integrated Management of Adolescent and Adult Illness, Interim Guidelines for First Level Facility Health Worker, WHO/ CDS/IMAI/2004.2. Geneva: WHO, 2004b.

World Trade Organization. Ministerial Declaration, Doha 2001. WT/ MIN(01)/DEC/1. 20 November 2001. Online document at: www.wto.org/english/thewto_e/minist_e/min01_e/mindecl_e.pdf. Accessed September 17, 2004.

Sangomas Step out of the Shadows

By Tom Nevin
African Business, June 2006

The doctor's note that lets employees take a few days off work is the latest glitch in efforts to bring together under one umbrella organisation South Africa's traditional healers and biomedical doctors.

Although the Traditional Health Practitioners' Act has already been signed into law, little real movement in applying the new legislation has been made, mainly due to the very wide gap waiting to be bridged between traditional and bio medicine. Economic, social and professional headaches abound. Just one of which is the issue of doctors' notes.

As it is, absenteeism punishes the South African economy by around R36bn ($6bn) each year in direct and indirect costs, including hiring and training additional staff. Prior to the new legislation only medical doctors, dentists and psychiatrists were empowered to issue notes that excused employees from work. The new law includes a much wider range of health professionals and workers with the same authority.

Labour specialist Andrew Levy says: "We now include physiotherapists, psychologists, naturopaths and many other paths you have never even heard of." Researcher Neesa Moodley, writing in *Business Report*, says South Africans spend about R250m on traditional healers each year and the act, gazetted in February last year, recognises more than 300,000 traditional healers.

According to Johnny Johnson, CEO of absenteeism management company CAM Solutions, once the act is viewed with the Basic Conditions of Employment Act, the implications for increased sick leave are obvious.

Associate attorney at Leppan Beech law firm, Ndumiso Voyi, says the thorniest aspect of the new act is that it is practically impossible to objectively verify findings by a traditional health practitioner, even by another traditional healer.

"If the health ministry fails to give the act teeth, the potential cost of this legislation to the economy could be catastrophic," he maintains, and calls for comprehensive regulations to support the act.

The South African department of health believes that around 70% of South Africans consult traditional healers in an industry the size of which can only be guessed at, but could be upwards of R400m a year. Around 60% of all babies born in South Africa are delivered by traditional birth attendants.

Professor Derek Hellenberg, deputy chairman of health policy at the South African Medical Association (SAMA) says tax collection in this vast alternative health sector is a major headache. "The Revenue Services fear millions, if not billions, of rands of taxable healers' income will slip through the cracks of cash payments, the method of settlement demanded by most healers."

David Phoshoko is one of a number of healers treating, counselling and consulting in GaRankuwa township north of Pretoria. Most of his patients can't afford much in the way of money, and so the greater percentage of his consultations is paid for in chickens, piece work, used clothing or other barter.

"We don't have hard and fast fee structures," says Phoshoko. "It all depends on the health and personal circumstances of each patient. How can you say that each condition is the same and we must charge the same? We are happy with fair payment, whatever it is. Goats are OK."

Away with "Witchcraft" Laws—Zim Judge

No other African country has taken such wide-reaching steps to bring the two health providers together as South Africa, although pressure is being brought on the Zimbabwe government to lift restrictions on traditional healing, still known there as "witchcraft", the term imposed by the British colonial government early last century. The latest urging to throw out the colonial law has come from a senior High Court judge in Bulawayo, Maphios Cheda.

"Many here retain strong beliefs in the healing power of spirit mediums—known as *nyangas* or witchdoctors—along with the role of ancestral rites in the nation's cultural life," he says. "The strongly-held conviction of belief in witchcraft and traditional healers cannot be wished away. Let us have amendments to the 100-year-old Witchcraft Suppression Act in keeping with the popular thinking and beliefs of the majority of the country."

He quotes estimates by the Zimbabwe National Traditional Healers' Association that at least 80% of Zimbabweans visit healers for treatment and consultation.

A fear that has kept many African governments from allowing traditional healers the same status as biomedical doctors is the additional spending state health services would have to foot, and the flood of patients referred by healers hospitals and clinics would have to accommodate.

A Meeting of Minds?

The South African Medical Association has been tracking the problem for the past 14 years, regularly updating its seminal study *Bridging the Gap: Potential for Healthcare Partnerships between African Traditional Healers and Biomedical Personnel*. It has always held the view that a nationally-legislated policy that accepted traditional healers as providers of healthcare was required, based on proficiency criteria.

It also called for a standardised core training programme in primary health biomedicine to enable traditional healers to work alongside biomedical personnel. At the same time, biomedical personnel would be required to take courses that explained the nature and methods of traditional healing, including community-based health education. Also recommended was the creation of a national drug formulary of traditional healing.

> Traditional healing methods play an important role in the treatment of illnesses perceived to be of supernatural origin.

The analysis focused on patient-healer relationship, types of healers, their training and role in the community, perceptions of traditional healers, therapeutic methods and attempts at collaboration. Data collected indicates points of both convergence and divergence between traditional healing and biomedicine.

The overriding aim of the review was to investigate the current and past role of African traditional healers in healthcare delivery and to make recommendations in respect of their potential in the South African healthcare system.

The distinction between natural and "supernatural" causes of illnesses was found to influence an individual's choice on whether to consult a traditional healer or a biomedical service. Traditional healing methods play an important role in the treatment of illnesses perceived to be of supernatural origin.

"More empirical research on traditional healing is required on two fronts" the study recommended. The first, to he undertaken by sociologists, psychologists and medical anthropologists, would examine the role played by applied ethnology, religion, culture and psychology in all aspects of medicine and the healing process as a whole. The second entails the more rational study of herbal remedies and is the concern of doctors, pharmacists, botanists and pharmacologists.

"The medical profession should be educated about traditional healing in an attempt to dispel misconceptions and suspicions" the report stated, adding that this could be achieved by SAMA encouraging its members to liaise with traditional healers and initiating cross referral of patients, by educating the medical profession through scientific journals and sessions on traditional healing at SAMA's annual conferences.

Dr Alan Smith, virologist at Durban's Albert Lithuli Hospital says not much progress is being made in a meeting of the minds. "Traditional healing is not specifically an African phenomenon; alternative healing methods are found worldwide. Inherently, people like to take care of themselves. They're suspicious of high-powered medicine."

Smith believes that if modern healthcare has lost anything, it's the mystique of medicine.

"Patients have lost that wonderful faith in their doctor," he says. "Fifty years ago doctors could not offer their patients much therapeutic aid, so it was really a matter of helping patients along until they healed themselves. Applying that to the context of Africa, traditional healers throughout the continent have long applied treatment of this kind. They basically had two types of therapy—one is the Sangoma who works somewhat like a parish priest who boosts your faith in yourself, and the other, the *Inyanga* would be the herbalist. Undoubtedly there's power in those ancient processes of healing and we have learnt, and are still learning a lot from them," he says.

V. U.S. Response to Africa's Health Care Crisis

Editor's Introduction

As the world's richest country and the only current superpower, the United States has been under pressure to respond to the global AIDS crisis and, specifically, to problematic issues throughout sub-Saharan Africa. The international response has been considerable, with many nongovernmental organizations establishing programs, such as the UN's Millienium Goals, to eradicated disease, poverty, and hunger. The United States has periodically sent aid in the past, but in 2003, under President George W. Bush, a permanent aid structure, President's Emergency Program for AIDS Relief (PEPFAR), was instituted. It was created to fight the pandemic on a global scale, but because of the high percentage of cases on the sub-Saharan continent, much of the funding has been allocated to help secure the health care system. Recently, for the upcoming budget, President Bush proposed increasing the budget for PEPFAR from $15 billion to $18.3 billion. This would make the United States the largest single contributor to an international health initiative, but some critics claim that the funds actually received are far below the promised level, while the situation in Africa continues to worsen.

In the chapter's first article, "Analysis of President George W. Bush's Emergency Plan for AIDS Relief in Sub-Saharan Africa and the Caribbean," Dr. Paul S. Zeitz describes the intentions outlined in the president's plan, but argues that it does not do enough to augment change. He points out that, despite the government's promise of an unprecedented amount for AIDS relief, much of that money has been taken from other programs, which leaves those areas to suffer. In the end Zeitz feels that the benefits of PEPFAR have been exaggerated.

In "Public-Private Partnerships to Enhance Delivery of AIDS Drugs," a State News Service released a detailed description of how a cooperation between public and private health care systems can help improve the situation in Africa. The article states that this collaboration will help deliver pharmaceuticals and medical supplies to the developing world, and as a part of PEPFAR, the State Department suggests that this partnership will help ensure a "robust lifeline" of supplies. To offer a counter argument to the State Department's claims, the fourth article, "Promises, Promises" by Erica Casriel, discusses the inadequacies of PEPFAR, lists the current administration's unfulfilled pledges, and offers alternative means of increasing help to the subcontinent. Balancing out this argument is the fourth article, a brief description of the money allocated to Harvard by the Bush administration to support the university's plan to increase in five years the number of people with HIV/AIDS who will be afforded treatment.

As evidenced by the previous articles, the funding that has received the most attention has been focused on the fight against the HIV/AIDS virus, and as a result, other areas have been neglected. In the last article of this chapter, "Fatal Inaction," Joshua Kurlantzick raises the subject of malaria and how the United States can help in its treatment. He argues for the use artemisinin, which is combined with other drugs for a malaria therapy known as ACT. At the moment this therapy, though proven effective, is rarely used because of its costliness. Kurlantzick presents a history of the drugs used to combat malaria and the disease's eventual resistance to those treatments, as well as examples of how aid from the United States has ebbed and flowed through the years. He concludes that so far, aid from the U.S. and international sources has been inadequate.

Analysis of President George W. Bush's Emergency Plan for AIDS Relief in Sub-Saharan Africa and the Caribbean*

BY PAUL S. ZEITZ** AND DAVID BRYDEN***
EMORY INTERNATIONAL LAW REVIEW, SUMMER 2003

> And to meet a severe and urgent crisis abroad, tonight I propose the Emergency Plan for AIDS Relief—a work of mercy beyond all current international efforts to help the people of Africa. This comprehensive plan will prevent 7 million new AIDS infections, treat at least 2 million people with life-extending drugs, and provide humane care for millions of people suffering from AIDS, and for children orphaned by AIDS.
>
> *—President George W. Bush, State of the Union Address, January 28, 2003*

Introduction

On January 28, 2003, during his State of the Union Address, President Bush announced a historic plan, "Emergency Plan for AIDS Relief in sub-Saharan Africa and the Caribbean."[1] This announcement marks a watershed moment in the global response to the AIDS pandemic.

The President is to be commended for putting forth a bold plan and featuring it so prominently in the single most important speech in the context of U.S. politics. That the President has chosen to announce this initiative while facing other foreign policy challenges is a testament to the power of the broad and diverse advocacy movement that has doggedly campaigned for a Presidential AIDS initiative for the past two years.

Our response to AIDS is, quite simply, a matter of life and death. It is critical that President Bush's newly stated commitment to stopping global AIDS be translated into new, supplementary resources as soon as possible. It is high time for the President's statements of compassion to be turned into real programs that save lives on the ground in Africa and other regions of the World.

---

* The views advocated in this Article are those of the authors.

** Executive Director, Global AIDS Alliance.

*** Communications Director, Global AIDS Alliance.

Dr. Paul S. Zeitz & David Bryden, *Analysis of President George W. Bush's Emergency Plan for AIDS Relief in Sub-Saharan Africa and the Caribbean,* 17 EMORY INT'L L. REV. 955 (2003)

In this report, we review the President's Plan and raise key concerns about it, based on currently available information and the fiscal year (FY) 2004 budget request.

I. KEY CONCERNS REGARDING THE PRESIDENT'S EMERGENCY PLAN FOR AIDS RELIEF

Based on the information currently available, the following key concerns should be addressed by the Administration:

A. Bush's Plan Will Be Phased-in Too Slowly

The President's FY 2004 budget requests only $450 million for new bilateral programs.[2] In addition, the Global Fund will only receive $200 million each year for the next six years—a straight-line of funding indicating that the President intends to slowly phase-in his program.[3] From a public health standpoint, this is inappropriate. The epidemic is expanding exponentially even while there is extensive underfunding of currently available programs.

There is a wide consensus among public health advocates that the U.S. government should contribute to the global AIDS programs based on the U.S. share of the global economy. Since the U.S. share of the global economy is 32.2%,[6] the U.S. share of the global AIDS programs ($10.5 billion per year in total) should be $3.5 billion.

PRESIDENT BUSH'S EMERGENCY PLAN FOR AIDS RELIEF						
(in US$ millions)	Baseline	FY04	FY05	FY06	FY07	FY08
ONGOING BILATERAL SPENDING						
USAID-HIV/AIDS	500	650	500	500	500	500
USAID-HIV/AIDS-other economic assistance	40	40	40	40	40	40
HHS	144	294	144	144	144	144
NEW AIDS SPENDING						
GLOBAL AIDS INITIATIVE		450[4]	1250	1800	2400	2600
GLOBAL FUND						
	200	200	200	200	200	200
TOTAL SPENDING		1634	2134	2684	3284	3484

B. Bush's Plan Undermines "Multilateral" Global Fund

President Bush's Plan will only provide $1 billion (10%) of the $10 billion of proposed new spending for the multilateral Global Fund to Fight AIDS, Tuberculosis and Malaria (the "Global Fund").[7]

The Global Fund's Financial Prospectus estimates that it needs $6.3 billion during 2003 and 2004 to fund proposals from countries,[8] in addition to the $2.2 billion needed to fund extensions of round one proposals a total of $8.5 billion.[9] Estimating the U.S. share based on its share of the global economy, we conclude that the United States should provide $2.9 billion from FY 2003 and FY 2004 resources to support the $8.5 billion need.[10] President Bush's Plan leaves the Global Fund without sufficient resources to support the scaling up of programs that are currently underway.

An additional problem arises with respect to management of the designated funds. Thus far, the President's Plan does not indicate which U.S. government agency will administer this effort or whether a new implementation structure is being considered to manage a majority of the funding. A large U.S. government investment should ideally be equally balanced between multilateral and bilateral programs, based on their respective comparative advantages.

C. Does Bush's Plan Really Add New Money in FY 2004?

The President's FY 2004 budget request indicates that the President is reducing spending in other key development areas, such as child immunization programs, to fund the global AIDS effort.[11] This appears to be a pattern; the President's FY 2002 budget request increased spending for global AIDS programs by cutting allocations for child survival programs and other development priorities. Cutting money from other effective programs to fund this Plan is counterproductive to addressing Africa's needs.

President Bush's Cut Funding for Child Survival and Other Health Program (in millions of US$)[12]			
Program	FY 2003 Funding	FY 2004 President's Request	Reduced Spending: FY 03 - FY 04
Child Survival/ Maternal Health	$303 USAID	$285 USAID	- $18
Infectious Diseases	$177.5 USAID	$104 USAID	- $74

D. Will Bush Use FY 2003 Funds To Support His Plan?

The President's FY 2003 Budget requested $1.65 billion for Global Fund AIDS programs.[13] In January 2003, a bipartisan coalition of Senators joined together during the negotiations for FY 2003 Omnibus Appropriations Bill to offer an amendment to increase the FY 2003 U.S. contribution to the Fund by $100 million and for bilateral programs by $80 million.[14]

President Bush has the opportunity to increase spending even beyond the Senate Amendment discussed above during the FY 2004 Omnibus Appropriations process or with an FY 2003 Emergency Supplemental Appropriation. The President has not yet signaled whether he supports this vitally important amendment in the Senate.

II. BUSH'S PLAN TARGETS TOO FEW HEAVILY AFFECTED COUNTRIES

The President's Emergency Plan for AIDS Relief will help only twelve (25%) of forty-eight sub-Saharan countries. These countries include Botswana, Cote d'Ivoire, Ethiopia, Kenya, Mozambique, Namibia, Nigeria, Rwanda, South Africa, Tanzania, Uganda, and Zambia.[15] Other key countries that require U.S. leadership include Malawi, Swaziland, Eritrea, Ghana, Mali, Burkina Faso, Democratic Republic of the Congo, Cameroon, Lesotho and Zimbabwe, among others. In the Caribbean, the President's Plan only addresses Guyana and Haiti.[16]

Despite the National Intelligence Council report, released in November of 2002, on the next wave of the epidemic, countries such as Russia, China, and India have been overlooked for increased funding.[17]

A. Will Bush's Plan Fully Address the Orphans' Crisis?

The U.S. government reports that there are currently fourteen million children orphaned by AIDS,[18] with a projected number of twenty-five million by 2010—the majority of these in sub-Saharan Africa.[19] Thus far, the President has not described any detailed commitment designed to address the needs of this group of affected people.

B. Bush's Plan Does Not Provide Debt Cancellation for Priority Countries

Nearly all of the countries prioritized in the President's Plan are burdened with unsustainable debt payments that undermine the capacity of their governments to effectively respond to the AIDS crisis or to combat poverty. In 2001, African governments paid $13.6 billion in debt servicing payments to the International Monetary Fund, the World Bank, and wealthy nation creditors.[20] This extraction of local resources directly undermines all efforts to combat AIDS. To ensure those U.S. investments under the President's Emergency Plan for AIDS Relief are matched with local resources, the President should incorporate debt cancellation into his plan.

C. Will Bush's Plan Support the Purchase of Generically Manufactured Drugs?

In the President's State of the Union address he referred to life-extending antiretroviral agents that cost less than $300 per year.[21] Procurement of drugs at this rate is only possible from generic manufacturers. While the Administration has stated that the new AIDS programs will support procurement of generically-manufactured antiretroviral drugs,[22] it is uncertain whether Congress will approve such purchases through U.S. government agencies. In contrast, the Global Fund has already adopted a policy which allows countries the option of procuring generic drugs.[23]

D. Will Bush's Plan Include Investment in Anti-Corruption Measures to Ensure a Return on Investment?

As no major partner is currently addressing accountability issues as part of the global HIV/AIDS response, we strongly recommend that the President's Plan identify, assess, and fully fund innovative strategies to ensure accountability of resources and to combat drug sector corruption so that U.S. taxpayers get a high return on their investment.

III. BUSH EXAGGERATES U.S. SUPPORT

The Bush Administration tends to exaggerate the U.S. contribution toward the global effort to fight AIDS by including what the U.S. spends on research programs.[24] The Global AIDS Alliance supports research, but the cost targets of the World Health Organization (WHO) and the United Nationsl Special Programme on HIV/AIDS (UNAIDS) for the global AIDS response excludes research—instead, this estimate is only for on-the-ground delivery of services. By including research programs in budget estimates, the Bush Administration exaggerates the U.S. contribution towards the WHO/UNAIDS program targets.

A. Fact Sheet on Global AIDS Funding

1. Cost of Global AIDS Response

Global experts from WHO and UNAIDS estimate that $10.5 billion per year is needed to fund a minimum package of currently available prevention, care and support, treatment with lifesaving medications, and a response to the burgeoning orphans crisis for people living in impoverished nations.[25] During 2002, UNAIDS estimated that approximately $3.0 billion from all sources was spent in poor countries, less than one-third of the estimated total global need.[26]

2. U.S. Spending for Global AIDS

There is a wide consensus among public health advocates that the U.S. Government should allocate $3.5 billion per year during 2003 for global AIDS programs, based on the U.S. proportion of the global economy. The President's FY 2003 Budget requests $1.65 billion for the Global Fund's AIDS programs.[27]

U.S. SPENDING ON GLOBAL AIDS DURING BUSH ADMINISTRATION

U.S. SPENDING ON GLOBAL HIV/AIDS (EXCLUDING RESEARCH)				
(in USD million)	FY 2002	FY 2003 Request	FY 2003 Senate	FY 2004 Request
BILATERAL[32]				
USAID	395	600	622	650
CDC	144	244	169	294
Other	40	40	50	40
Subtotal Bilateral	579	884	841	984
GLOBAL FUND[33]				
	200	200	300–400	200
TOTAL	779	1084	1141–1241	1184

3. Total Needs for the Global Fund to Fight AIDS, Tuberculosis, and Malaria

Since accepting its first pledges in 2001, the Global Fund has rapidly garnered the trust of donors and recipients as one of the most effective implementing tools available for the disbursement of resources based on country needs. In its first round of grants awarded in June of 2002, the Global Fund awarded $616 million over two years to projects in forty countries.[28] In 2003, the Global Fund awarded another $866 million for new projects in sixty countries.[29]

According to the Global Fund's Financial Prospectus, in order to finance all of the highest quality applications in the next rounds, it will need a total of at least $6.3 billion over 2003-2004.[30] The Fund has asked the United States for between $2.5 and $3.0 billion of this total, a contribution calculated using the relative GDP of the United States.[31] Numerous well-thought-out applications will be turned away unless new pledges are made immediately.

Footnotes

1. President George W. Bush, State of the Union Address (Jan. 28, 2003), *available at* http://www.whitehouse.gov/news/releases/2003/01/20030128-19.html (last visited Aug. 27, 2003).

2. Executive Office of the President of the United States, Budget of the United States Government, Fiscal Year 2004, at 216 (2004) [hereinafter Budget: FY 2004], *available at:* http://www.whitehouse.gov/omb/budget/fy2004/pdf/budget.pdf (last visited Aug. 27, 2003).

3. *Id.* at 120.

4. Budget: FY 2004, *supra note* 2, at 216.

5. Global Fund Pledges, June 10, 2003, http://www.aidspan.org/gfo/does/gfo56.xls (last visited Aug. 27, 2003).

6. *See* The World Bank, World Development Indicators Database: Total GDP 2002 (2003), *available at* http://www.worldbank.org/data/databytopic/GDP.pff (last visited Aug. 27, 2003).

7. BUDGET: FY 2004, *supra* note 2, at 216.

8. The Global Fund to Fight AIDS, Tuberculosis & Malaria, Global Fund Secretariat, *Financial Prospectus: Status and Forecasts for Resource Mobilization*, Jan. 2003, at 1 [hereinafter *Financial Prospectus*], *available at* http://www.aidspan.org(gfo/docstgfo37.pdf (last visited Aug. 27, 2003).

9. *See* The Global Fund to Fight AIDS, Tuberculosis & Malaria, Secretariat Discussion Paper, *Discussion Document on the Development of a Comprehensive Policy for Approving & Funding Grants*, June 5, 2003, at para. 19 (stating that no funds had been reserved for extensions of successful Round One programs), http://www.globalfundatm.org/fifthboardmeeting/filesgfb55a.pdf (last visited Aug. 27, 2003).

10. *NEWS: Feachem on the Record*, GLOBAL FUND OBSERVER NEWSLETTER (The Global Fund to Fight AIDS, Tuberculosis and Malaria, Geneva, Switzerland), Jan. 10, 2003, at 4, *available at* http//www.aidspan.org/gfo/archives/newsletter/issue2.pdf (last visited Aug. 27, 2003)

11. Lou Chibbaro, Jr., *Bush Boosts AIDS Funding, but Cuts HIV Prevention: Budget Draws Mixed Reviews from Gay, AIDS Advocacy Groups*, THE WASHINGTON BLADE, Feb. 7, 2003, *at* http://www.aegia.com/news/wb/2003/WB030202.html (last visited Aug. 27, 2003).

12. Global Health Council, Global Health Funding, http:/twww.globalhealth.org/ view_top.php3?id=172 (last visited Aug. 27, 2003).

13. *Global AIDS. An Economic and Moral Imperative*, June 6, 2003, http:/www.globalhealth.gov/102GlobFund.rtf (last visited Aug. 27, 2003).

14. Press Release, Senator Dick Durbin, Global AIDS Funding Included in Federal Spending Bill (Jan. 23, 2003) (cosponsoring the Senate bill were Senators Durbin and DeWine), *available at* http://durbin.senate.gov/~durbin/new200l/press/2003/01/2003123D55.html (last visited Aug. 27, 2003).

15. U.S. State Dep't, *The President's Emergency Plan for AIDS Relief*, Jan. 29, 2003, *available at* http://www.state.gov/p/af/rls/fs/17033.htm (last visited Aug. 27, 2003).

16. *Id.*

17. NAT'L INTELLIGENCE COUNCIL, CENTRAL INTELLIGENCE AGENCY, THE NEXT WAVE OF HIV/AIDS: NIGERIA, ETHIOPIA, RUSSIA, INDIA, AND CHINA, *passim* (2002), *available at* http://www.cia.gov/nietpubs/other_products/ICA%20HlV-AIDS%20unclassified%20092302POSTGERBER.htm (last visited Aug. 27, 2003).

18. Press Release, Office of the Press Secretary, Fact Sheet: The President's Emergency Plan for AIDS Relief (Jan. 29, 2003), *available at* http://www.whitehouse.gov/news/releases/2003/01/20030129-1.html (last visited Aug. 27, 2003).

19. USAID ET AL., CHILDREN ON THE BRINK 2002, at 1 (2002), *available at* http://www.unaids.org/barcelona/presskit/childrenonthebrink.html (last visited Aug. 27, 2003).

20. *See* THE WORLD BANK, GLOBAL DEVELOPMENT FINANCE 2001, at 254 (2001), *available at* http://www.worldbank.org/prospectst/gdf200l/vol1-pdf/mna.pdf (last visited Aug. 27, 2003).

21. Bush, *supra* note 1.

22. *See* Press Release, Office of the Press Secretary, *supra* note 18.

23. *See* The Global Fund to Fight AIDS, Tuberculosis and Malaria, *Principles*, http://www.globalfundatm.org/principles.html (last visited Aug. 27, 2003) (stating that the Global Fund will support proposals that "encourage efforts to make quality drugs and products available at the lowest possible prices for those in need").

24. *See* President George W. Bush, Remarks on Global and Domestic HIV/AIDS (Jan. 31, 2003), *available at* http://www.whitehouse.gov/news/releases/2003/0l/20030131-4.html (last visited Aug. 27, 2003).

25. Press Release, UNAIDS, New Figures Show AIDS Under-Resources (Oct. 10, 2002), *available at* http://www.unaids.org/whatsnew/press/eng/pressarc02/GlobalFund101002_en.html (last visited Aug. 27, 2003).

26. Peter Piot, Editorial, *In Poor Nations, a New Will to Fight AIDS*, N.Y. TIMES, July 3, 2002, at 23A.

27. *Global AIDS. An Economic and Moral Imperative, supra* note 13.

28. *Financial Prospectus, supra* note 8, at 2.

29. *Id.* at 4.

30. *Id.*

31. *NEWS: Feachem on the Record, supra* note 10, at 4.

32. RAYMOND W. COPSON, CONGRESSIONAL RESEARCH SERVICE, LIBRARY OF CONGRESS, HIV/AIDS INTERNATIONAL PROGRAMS: APPRORIATIONS, FY2002–FY2004, at CRS-2 (2004).

33. *Global Fund Pledges,* June 10, 2003, http://www.aidspan.org/gfo/docs/gfo56.xls (last visited Aug. 27, 2003).

Public-Private Partnership to Enhance Delivery of AIDS Drugs

USINFO.STATE.GOV, SEPTEMBER 28, 2005

Building an improved system for delivering pharmaceuticals and medical supplies to the developing world is the goal of a public-private partnership announced by the U.S. Agency for International Development (USAID) September 27.

"By building human and institutional supply chain capacity in developing countries, this system will help rapidly expand prevention, care and treatment for people living with and affected by HIV/AIDS," USAID Administrator Andrew Natsios said.

The partnership involves 15 separate U.S. and African companies and groups specializing in various services and skills critical to building a system to move medical supplies and drugs efficiently and reliably.

Drug delivery specialists, business consultants, information technology specialists and nongovernmental organizations with experience in Africa will participate in building this new system, according to USAID press materials.

The partnership is created as part of the five-year, $15 billion President's Emergency Plan for AIDS Relief, which is helping combat the epidemic in more than 100 nations around the world, with a special focus on 15 nations suffering the world's greatest disease burden.

Following are USAID press materials explaining the initiative:

Under the President's Emergency Plan for AIDS Relief, USAID Announces Contract to Swiftly Deliver Lifesaving Medicines and Supplies to Developing Countries

Consortium of 15 Institutions to Implement Award

September 27, 2005

Today, the President's Emergency Plan for AIDS Relief, through the U.S. Agency for International Development, announced a contract to strengthen the lifeline of essential drugs and supplies for people living with or affected by HIV/AIDS and other infectious diseases in developing countries. The winning team is called The Partnership for Supply Chain Management (the Partnership) and is a

Source: U.S. Department of State. Material in the public domain.

leading consortium of 15 separate institutions from the private sector, non-profit and faith-based community, and is well connected to existing delivery and purchasing systems in the developing world.

The award was determined by an interagency selection panel, half of which included representatives from USAID, as well as representatives from the U.S. Department of Health and Human Services and the U.S. Department of Defense. The panel's overall decision was unanimous.

Designed by an expert interagency team headed by the Office of the U.S. Global AIDS Coordinator, SCMS further advances the Emergency Plan's initial strategy for an effective and accountable supply chain system to help developing countries rapidly scale-up prevention, care and treatment programs. Based on the winning proposal, the contract funds up to $77 million in system operating expenses and technical assistance over the first three years. The drugs and supplies handled by the system could total $500 million or more over that same period. The contract will be responsive to requests from countries and programs in the field and will be adjusted accordingly.

Specifically, SCMS will provide one stop shopping for programs to obtain important HIV/AIDS-related products. These will include facilitating the purchase of lifesaving antiretroviral drugs; drugs for opportunistic infections such as tuberculosis; quality laboratory materials such as rapid test kits; and supplies like gowns, gloves, injection equipment, cleaning and sterilization items.

"The U.S. government believes that without local, sustainable capacity, nations cannot fully 'own' the fight they must lead against HIV/AIDS. This capacity is a prerequisite for national programs that achieve results, monitor and evaluate their activities, and sustain their responses for the long-term," said Randall L. Tobias, the U.S. Global AIDS Coordinator.

Implemented by USAID's new Division of Supply Chain Management within the Bureau for Global Health, SCMS will establish a transparent and accountable system for the secure and reliable supply of high-quality, low-cost products. Critical components of the supply chain include:

- Developing and maintaining a competitive and transparent procurement system, including forecasting future need and leverage volume purchasing to achieve significant reductions in the current cost of supplies;

- Establishing a quality assurance plan to manage documentation and ensure quality of supplies;

- Providing freight forwarding and warehousing services to facilitate consolidation and shipping from manufacturers worldwide;

- Establishing in-country support teams to provide the highly complex technical assistance needed to improve existing programs;

- Developing Management Information Systems to track supplies provided through SCMS by estimating needs by recipient programs, financial accounts by country and funding source, production and warehouse stock levels, and the status of all shipments in-transit.

"By building human and institutional supply chain capacity in developing countries, this system will help rapidly expand prevention, care, and treatment for people living with and affected by HIV/AIDS," USAID Administrator Andrew S. Natsios said.

The Partnership for Supply Chain Management includes:

- Affordable Medicines for Africa—Johannesburg, South Africa

- AMFA Foundation—St. Charles, Ill.

- Booz Allen Hamilton—McLean, Va.

- Crown Agents Consultancy, Inc.—Washington, DC

- Fuel Logistics Group (Pty) Ltd.—Sandton, South Africa

- International Dispensary Association—Amsterdam, Netherlands

- JSI Research and Training Institute, Inc.—Boston, Mass.

- Management Sciences for Health, Inc.— Boston, Mass.

- The Manoff Group, Inc.—Washington, DC

- MAP International—Brunswick, Ga.

- The North-West University—Potchefstroom, South Africa

- Northrop Grumman Information Technology—McLean, Va.

- Program for Appropriate Technology in Health—Seattle, Wash.

- UPS Supply Chain Solutions[SM]—Atlanta, Ga.

- Voxiva, Inc.—Washington, DC

The President's Emergency Plan for AIDS Relief is a five-year, $15 billion, multifaceted approach to combating HIV/AIDS, including bilateral programs in more than 100 countries around the world. As of March 2005, the Emergency Plan has supported anti-retroviral treatment for more than 235,000 men, women and children through bilateral programs in 15 of the most afflicted countries in Africa, Asia and the Caribbean. More than 230,000 of those being supported live in sub-Saharan Africa. The U.S. continues to support treatment for more people than any other donor in the world.

Leadership Through Compassionate Action: A New "Partnership for Supply Chain Management"

September 27, 2005

The Rationale

Comprehensive HIV/AIDS programs that are sustained for the long-term require a continuous inflow of essential medicines and supplies. In most developing countries, limited health systems capacity is a major challenge to providing the appropriate health care many urgently need. In concert with in-country partners, the Bush Administration is leading the world in building the necessary infrastructure to fight the global pandemic of HIV/AIDS. The President's Emergency Plan for AIDS Relief, through its new Partnership for Supply Chain Management (the Partnership), will strengthen systems to deliver an uninterrupted supply of high-quality, lost-cost products that will flow through a transparent, accountable system.

The Purpose

The winning consortium—unprecedented in its magnitude and scope—will help deliver essential lifesaving medicines to the front lines of U.S. government HIV/AIDS programs. The Partnership will ensure a healthy, robust lifeline of continuous drugs and supplies that are safe, secure, reliable and sustainable. These will include supporting the purchase of lifesaving antiretroviral drugs (including low-cost generic ARVs tentatively approved by the U.S. Food and Drug Administration); drugs for opportunistic infections such as tuberculosis; quality laboratory materials such as rapid test kits; and supplies like gowns, gloves, injection equipment, cleaning and sterilization items. Based on the winning proposal, the contract funds up to $77 million in system operating expenses and technical assistance over the first three years. The drugs and supplies handled by the system could total $500 million or more over that same period. The contract will be responsive to requests from countries and programs in the field and will be adjusted accordingly.

The Approach

At the heart of the President's Emergency Plan is its work with partners in host nations in support of their respective national strategies on HIV/AIDS. The Partnership will devise and implement technical solutions that will transform the way in which HIV/AIDS drugs and supplies reach the people who need them most. The Partnership will strengthen current national supply chain mechanisms, and will implement a fully functional pharmaceutical supply chain for the President's Emergency Plan, working at three levels:

- National: the public and private organizations, programs, services and structures in countries served by the President's Emergency Plan;

- Regional: the services and structures for warehousing and supply distribution at the regional level, using existing service providers;

- Global: activities and services organized predominantly at the global level, including procurement, global logistics, quality assurance, external communications, headquarters-level coordination and program management.

The Components

The President's Emergency Plan Partnership will not build parallel systems; it will be additive and complementary to existing supply chain efforts in the field. It is intended to "fill in the gaps" where supply chain services are needed the most. The supply chain will:

- Develop and maintain a competitive and transparent procurement system, including forecasting future need and leveraging volume purchasing to achieve significant reductions in the current costs of commodities.

- Establish a quality assurance plan to manage documentation and ensure quality of commodities.

- Provide freight forwarding and warehousing services to facilitate consolidation and shipping from manufacturers worldwide.

- Establish in-country support teams to provide the highly complex technical assistance needed to improve existing programs.

- Develop Management Information Systems (MIS) to track the commodities provided through this agreement by estimating needs by recipient programs, financial accounts by country and funding source, production and warehouse stock levels, and the status of all shipments in-transit.

Participation

Participation in the Partnership is voluntary and services can be selectively utilized depending on the needs of the country and program. In those countries where existing supply chains are working well, the Partnership will be available as an option to "fill in the gaps" and monitor key steps in the supply chain process.

Non-ARV Drugs

The Partnership will support the purchase of non-ARV drugs that are needed for HIV/AIDS patients, including drugs for opportunistic infections, sexually transmitted infections, tuberculosis and some anti-malarial drugs. In addition, drugs needed for home and palliative care of HIV/AIDS patients will be purchased.

About the Partnership

The Partnership for Supply Chain Management is a non-profit organization established in 2005 by two international leaders in supply chain management for drugs and other public health commodities in developing countries—JSI Research and Training (JSI), and Management Sciences for Health (MSH). The Partnership includes 13 other organizations, each one offering unique capabilities that will ensure that high-quality antiretroviral drugs, HIV tests, and other supplies for treating HIV/AIDS are available to the people-patients, clinicians, laboratory technicians, and others—who need them.

- Affordable Medicines for Africa (AMFA) is a South African-based not-for-gain organization that has developed a rapid response supply chain management system to provide African health care providers with African manufactured medicines under African quality control through African distribution channels. AMFA provides a comprehensive and consistent supply of 230 high-quality, affordable, essential medicines and medical supplies to 13 African countries.

- AMFA Foundation is a U.S.-based nonprofit international Christian service organization whose goal is to provide affordable medicines for all in Africa, Asia, and the Americas. The Foundation helps create sustainable programs and innovative approaches to ensure Christian health care professionals in charitable hospitals and clinics can access high-quality, affordable medicines and supplies in a way that promotes the local economy in developing countries.

- Booz Allen Hamilton is a global strategy and technology consulting firm that works with clients across all major industries and for government agencies around the world to provide best-in-class strategic sourcing, manufacturing strategy, and techniques for managing complexity, while building self-sustaining capabilities that ensure these results endure. Booz Allen has implemented programs to strengthen institutional capacity in India, South America, and Africa.

- Crown Agents Consultancy, Inc., specializes in procurement services and supporting and strengthening supply chains, working with public and private sectors in more than 100 countries, as well as with international agencies. Crown Agents conducts ARV procurement for JSI's DELIVER project, serving President's Plan programs in Tanzania and Zambia, and is one of the largest worldwide purchasers of HIV/AIDS test kits.

- Fuel Logistics Group (Pty) Ltd., one of South Africa's top Black Economic Empowerment companies, has provided specialist pharmaceutical distribution services for almost 25 years. As a leading supply chain management corporation, Fuel's seven service-focused business units provide secure warehousing, inventory management, distribution, and IT services to more than 350 multinational customers and over 1,500 local commercial enterprises throughout southern Africa.

- International Dispensary Association (IDA) is the leader in the provision of essential medicines and related supplies to developing counties. With broad experience in procurement of pharmaceuticals and medical supplies, IDA offers qualified staff for vendor's audit and the selection of manufacturers, state-of-the-art quality assurance and quality control processes for pharmaceuticals, and deep knowledge and experience in international drug regulatory affairs. In addition, IDA is expert in pharmaceutical wholesaling, warehousing, and distribution to a broad variety of destinations.

- JSI Research and Training Institute, Inc. (JSI) is dedicated to improving the health of individuals and communities in the United States and around the world. Founded in 1978 and having implemented projects in 84 countries since that time, JSI assists developing country governments, donor agencies, nongovernmental organizations, and private companies in strengthening health systems. Through the USAID-funded DELIVER project and related supply chain contracts, JSI helps to ensure the availability of health supplies by strengthening systems, training people to manage those systems, helping governments develop policies that support commodity security, and mobilizing financing for essential health commodities.

- Management Sciences for Health, Inc. (MSH), a nonprofit organization with more than 1,000 staff worldwide, promotes a comprehensive response to public health issues, such as HIV/AIDS, through integrated technical assistance aimed at improving the management of people, medicines, money, and systems. MSH drug management professionals work with host country partners to implement innovative systems for high quality medicines. MSH currently manages two major pharmaceutical management programs that work in Emergency Plan focus countries: the Rational Pharmaceutical Management Plus cooperative agreement (RPM+) and Strategies for Enhancing Access to Medicines (SEAM).

- The Manoff Group, Inc. is a woman-owned small business that provides assistance in communications and behavior-centered planning, management and evaluations for health, nutrition, and population projects. The firm has been at the forefront of social marketing development since it first applied commercial marketing techniques to social programs in India in 1967. Since then, The Manoff Group has brought innovations in qualitative research methods, communication strategies, media planning and the creation of training materials to health, family planning, environment and nutrition programs around the globe.

- MAP International, founded 50 years ago, is a world leader in receipt and distribution of donated medicines and medical supplies for the developing world. With a staff of 130 working on three continents, this nonprofit relief and development agency provides essential medicines through a network of hospitals, clinics and community/relief center dispensaries in more than 120 countries. MAP has successfully distributed over $1.8 billion worth of medicines and medical supplies since its founding.

- The North-West University, part of South Africa's premier university system, comprises the drug analytical and development experience of the NWU Research Institute of Industrial Pharmacy and the Center for Quality Assurance of Medicines (CENQAM), among others. A designated WHO Collaborating Center for quality assurance (QA), CENQAM has been a regional leader in QA and training since 1994.

- Northrop Grumman Information Technology is the largest systems integrator serving the needs of the USG, including USAID and each of the funding agencies that supports the President's Plan. Northrop Grumman currently manages a $600 million contract providing IT support to the Centers for Disease Control.

- Program for Appropriate Technology in Health (PATH), founded in 1977, is an international nonprofit organization that creates sustainable, culturally relevant solutions, enabling communities worldwide to break longstanding cycles of poor health. By collaborating with diverse public- and private-sector partners, PATH helps provide appropriate health technologies and vital strategies that change the way people think and act. PATH's experience in global health spans the fields of reproductive health, vaccines and immunization, HIV/AIDS, tuberculosis, and maternal and child health and nutrition.

- UPS Supply Chain Solutions℠ has over 100 years of experience in providing specialized transportation and logistics services, with proven capabilities and global reach in 200 countries and territories worldwide. UPS is able to provide a variety of value-added supply chain services focusing on the movement of heavy-weight freight for commercial, industrial, and government customers worldwide. Voxiva is a U.S.-based small business that provides practical and innovative information and communications solutions to improve public health programs in the developing world. Voxiva has provided governments and agencies with affordable tools to conduct real-time disease surveillance, respond to and control disease outbreaks, manage and evaluate health programs, and track critical supplies.

President's Emergency Plan for AIDS Relief Summary

The President's Emergency Plan for AIDS Relief is a five-year, $15 billion, multifaceted approach to combating HIV/AIDS, including bilateral programs in more than 100 countries around the world. As of March 2005, the Emergency Plan has supported anti-retroviral treatment for more than 235,000 men, women and children through bilateral programs in 15 of the most afflicted countries in Africa, Asia and the Caribbean. More than 230,000 of those being supported live in sub-Saharan Africa. The U.S. continues to support treatment for more people than any other donor in the world.

US$1.5 BILLION SCHEME CREATES MARKET FOR VACCINES

BY TALENT NGANDWE
SCIDEV.NET, FEBRUARY 12, 2007

A US$1.5 billion scheme is set to accelerate the development and availability of new vaccines for neglected diseases.

The Advance Market Commitments for Vaccines (AMC) scheme launched last week (9 February) with a pilot project targeting vaccines against pneumoccoccal disease.

The project will subsidise poor countries' vaccine purchases, guaranteeing the purchase and giving vaccine makers the confidence to develop new treatments and build enough production capacity to satisfy global demand.

It will run for 7–10 years and include provisions to ensure a long-term sustainable supply and price for the poorest countries.

Pneumoccoccal disease kills about 1.6 million people every year. By speeding the research and development process for vaccines, the project could save the lives of 5.4 million children in the developing world by 2030.

Executive secretary of the GAVI Alliance, Julian Lob-Levyt, said an early version of a pneumoccoccal vaccine is showing widespread success in developed countries.

But he said manufacturers lack the capacity to provide a vaccine well suited to developing countries on a large scale.

"We expect that new pneumoccoccal vaccines will reach developing countries by 2010, at least 10 years earlier than if the AMC were not available," said Lob-Levyt.

Vernon Mwaanga, Zambia's chief government spokesperson welcomed the scheme, which would bring relief to developing countries that cannot afford to buy expensive vaccines.

He urged the AMC to extend the programme to other diseases if this pilot proves successful.

AMC is a partnership between the Bill and Melinda Gates Foundation and five developed countries—Canada, Italy, Norway, Russia and the United Kingdom.

It will be overseen by an independent assessment committee, which will set up and monitor standards for the vaccines.

The World Health Organization will help identify promising vaccines to target, and assess their quality, safety and effectiveness. The GAVI Alliance and the World Bank will also help with the initiative's planning and financial administration.

A total of US$1.5 billion has been committed to the project so far.

Article by Talent Ngandwe from SciDev.Net, www.scidev.net, February 12, 2007. Copyright © SciDev.Net. Reprinted with permission.

Promises, Promises

By Erika Casriel
The American Prospect, August 2004

At the June 2003 G8 Summit in Evian, France, President George W. Bush met with the other heads of state at a private dinner. There, according to sources close to two dinner guests, he promised the Europeans that if they gave $1 billion to a new joint AIDS fund, he would match it. But by July, Bush was urging Congress to supply no more than $200 million for the Global Fund to Fight AIDS, Tuberculosis and Malaria. "I think everybody felt fooled," says a Global Fund official.

Ultimately, Congress rebelled, increasing the U.S. contribution to the Global Fund to $547 million, but Bush has again budgeted only $200 million for the Global Fund in 2005. The president fails to mention these skirmishes when he claims that his administration is leading the world in the war on AIDS.

While it's true that the United States is contributing more than any other single country, the president has repeatedly overstated the U.S. financial commitment. Moreover, he has damaged the U.S alliance with international agencies fighting AIDS. Rather than join the world's AIDS battle plan—with the Global Fund as financier and monitor, the World Health Organization as technical adviser, and the Joint United Nations Programme on HIV/AIDS (UNAIDS) as coordinator—Bush has created his own controversial strategy with a separate set of rules for his 15 recipient countries. "At this point, the Bush plan is hurting more than it's helping," says Paul Zeitz, director of the Global AIDS Alliance, an advocacy group.

Bush announced that program, known as the President's Emergency Plan for AIDS Relief (PEPFAR), in his 2003 State of the Union address, when he promised a $15 billion, five-year mission to combat AIDS in Africa and the Caribbean. In a May 2003 ceremony with African ambassadors at the U.S. State Department, Bush signed a bill authorizing $3 billion in spending for the first year; during his July 2003 trip to Africa, the president spoke of the coming "$15 billion." His African audiences assumed that $3 billion would be sent in the first year, but the 2004 budget to fight global AIDS amounted to only $2 billion. With the price of AIDS drugs dropping, the billion-dollar shortfall translates into thousands of untreated AIDS patients.

The first round of PEPFAR funding wasn't distributed until February of this year; recipients included Save the Children and Harvard and Columbia universities. The plan covers 12 countries in Africa, two in the Caribbean, and Vietnam. AIDS experts applaud Randall Tobias, who was confirmed last fall in the new State Department post of global AIDS coordinator, for sending U.S. money out quickly after he got it. But they question whether PEPFAR will meet even its first-year goal of putting 201,000 people on anti-retroviral drugs.

"Many [African] health ministers are worried," says Celina Shocken, adviser to the HIV/AIDS minister of Rwanda, "that the first assessments will show very little progress in getting people on treatment." In May, the Council on Foreign Relations, a nonpartisan group, and the Milbank Memorial Fund, a nonpartisan health-policy foundation, published a report warning that PEPFAR is undefunded and doesn't emphasize local public-health systems, so that "five years from now . . . PEPFAR investment into programs directed to HIV/AIDS may fail to achieve its goals."

Bush's unwillingness to contribute fully both to his own program and to international efforts is consistent with his record: According to a 1999 Salon story, while in Texas, Bush was the only governor who did not participate in a campaign by the nonprofit organization Children Uniting Nations, which seeks to help Africans suffering from AIDS. Then, in March 2002, retiring Senator Jesse Helms of North Carolina called for $500 million to be disbursed that summer for drugs to help HIV-positive pregnant women in Africa avoid transmitting the virus to their babies. That summer, while Helms was in and out of the hospital, the White Housenegotiated the emergency AIDS funding from $500 million down to $200 million, which Congress approved. But Bush declined to release that money, announcing that he would instead request funding—in future fiscal years—for the prevention of HIV transmission from mother to child. As of this March, the United States had contracted out only $134 million for that program.

In January 2003, Bush finally called the AIDS epidemic an emergency, but it would be 13 months until $350 million was released. "Four and a half million people have died since Bush's announcement, and 10 million have died since he became president," says Paul Zeitz. "And in that time the U.S. has gotten about 1,000 people on treatment."

But the funding shortcomings and slow response are only part of the problem: Another obstacle, as with nearly every other global effort, is the Bush administration's insistence on working alone. In the case of AIDS, Bush has kept his distance from the Global Fund and leading AIDS agencies because they promote a "bottom-up" approach, meaning local stakeholders—including government, businesses, and community groups—meet and develop a plan to scale up their country's public-health system. The White House, on the other hand, is trying to create an AIDS program that is managed from inside the Beltway. And the reason for that is almost entirely ideological. When it comes to how to prevent and treat AIDS, Bush's positions are driven by the "pro-family" agenda of the American right, putting the White House and the global AIDS community into open debate.

To begin with, international agencies and the U.S. government can't even agree on whether condoms are essential to preventing the spread of AIDS. Speaking at a recent dinner in Berlin sponsored by the Global Business Coalition on HIV/AIDS, Tobias reflected the White House view when he said, "Statistics show that condoms really have not been very effective," adding that "it's been the principal prevention device for the last 20 years, and I think one needs only to look at what's happening with the infection rates in the world to recognize that has not been working." Under PEPFAR, condoms will be distributed only to unspecified "high-risk" groups.

But public-health experts counter that the rise of HIV is not a consequence of the focus on condoms, but rather of inadequate government attention to HIV prevention more generally. In the 1990s, Uganda was able to limit the spread of HIV through an intensive "ABC" campaign asking people to "Abstain, Be faithful, or use Condoms." While Bush officials point to Uganda's "A" as a model for other African programs, studies of Uganda's success—most recently

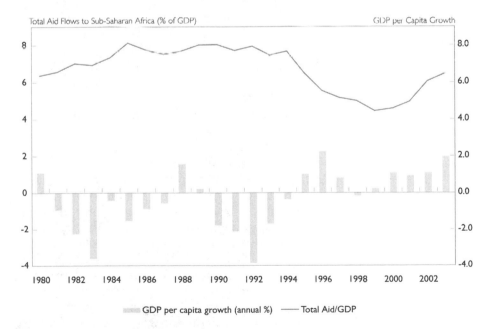

Aid and Economic Growth in Sub-Saharan Africa

GDP per capita growth (annual %) ——— Total Aid/GDP

Sources: World Bank, *World Development Indicators Online*, available at *www.worldbank.org/data*; Organisation for Economic Co-operation and Development, *International Development Statistics*, available at *http://www.oecd.org/dataoecd/50/17/5037721.htm*

in the April 30 issue of *Science* magazine—have shown that increased condom use in Uganda, in conjunction with a measured reduction in sexual partners, or "zero-grazing," as it was called, helped reduce the number of infections there.

Dr. Philippe Talavera, head of Obetja Yehinga, a public-health education campaign in Namibia, expects to see his group's U.S. funding (which had begun before PEPFAR) cut or eliminated because it brings up condom use with young people. "We were told that the money was to be subject to conditions," he wrote in an e-mail in response to questions for this article. "Condoms were to be promoted only with the high-risk groups (military, truck drivers, sex workers, drug addicts). This definition might work in the [United] States, but in a country where the prevalence is 22.5 [percent], everybody engaging in sexual activities has to be considered at risk."

Jodi Jacobson, executive director of the Center for Health and Gender Equity, a reproductive- and sexual-health group, says that U.S. officials and grant recipients "have told us that in three separate U.S. missions [in Africa], people are being told not to include any requests for condoms in their . . . operational strategies."

Another issue that splits the White House from the AIDS-relief community is abortion. Soon after his inauguration, Bush reinstated the "Mexico City Policy," also known as the global gag rule, which had been in effect under Presidents Ronald Reagan and George Bush Senior. Under these restrictions, foreign nongovernmental organizations receiving U.S. government funding must agree not to provide counseling or referral for abortion or perform abortions except in cases of rape, incest, or life-threatening illness. This policy has impeded the fight against AIDS by forcing the closure of many clinics. For example, the Kenya affiliate of Marie Stopes International, a reproductive-health-services group, had to shut down several clinics, including one that served 400 women a month in the province with the highest HIV prevalence rate in the country. In Ghana, the Planned Parenthood Association was forced to reduce not only family-planning services but also voluntary HIV testing and counseling for nearly 700,000 clients.

Bush's "pro-family" agenda is clear in his approach to grant giving as well. The United States is expected to invest about $180 million in abstinence-only-until-marriage programs—which don't discuss condoms or other forms of contraception—through PEPFAR in 2005. What's more, the Bush administration appears to be encouraging evangelical groups with no Africa experience to seek grants. In a conference with applicants, Dr. Anne Peterson, an administrator at the U.S. Agency for International Development, said that a "new partners' fund" has been set aside "for groups who've not ever worked with the U.S. government." According to a source close to the White House, this fund is intended to help American faith-based organizations seeking PEPFAR money. Bush has met with religious leaders at the White House about the HIV-prevention campaign in

Africa, and Tobias was the keynote speaker at a conference in November on PEPFAR and faith-based initiatives. At an earlier, similar meeting of Christian groups, Senator Rick Santorum said in a speech, "I, again, want to call on you to take advantage of this funding opportunity."

This emphasis on faith-based organizations has resulted in the exclusion of nonsectarian groups like the African Services Committee, which runs an HIV-testing center in Addis Ababa, Ethiopia, and sends outreach workers to urban outdoor markets. U.S. officials have praised the project, but when the committee tried to get U.S. financial help, the same officials were unresponsive. Kim Nichols, co-executive director of the African Services Committee, says, "[Faith-based organizations] seem to be getting all the attention."

The final point of tension between the administration and international public-health agencies is generic AIDS drugs. For three years, AIDS doctors in India and Africa have prescribed a single pill that contains three generic versions of brand-name anti-retroviral drugs. This allows AIDS patients to take two pills a day instead of six. "We know that patient convenience is one of the key factors in HIV/AIDS management," notes Dr. Jaideep Gogtay, chief medical adviser of the Indian company Cipla, one of two firms that produces these pills. (Cipla supplies the United States with a variety of generic drugs, but not anti-retrovirals, which are still under patent here.)

The generic, two-pill-a-day regime has proven to be as successful as brand-name drugs in clinical outcomes in current programs; the World Health Organization has sanctioned the drugs through a formal prequalification process; the Global Fund permits the purchase of World Health Organization–approved drugs; and they are licensed by the regulatory authorities of many countries in Africa that are already using them. They cost between $140 and $270 per patient per year, as compared with a discounted brand-name triple-combination course of treatment, which costs more than $500 per year, according to Doctors Without Borders.

But one of Tobias' first actions was to begin question the safety of the generic drugs. Then he made clear that PEPFAR funds could not be used to purchase them. "Maybe these drugs are safe and effective," he told a group of African journalists. "Maybe they aren't. Nobody really knows." PEPFAR grantees have thus been delayed in buying the generics. Faced with global outcry, including protest letters from African health ministers and bipartisan pressure from Congress, Tobias—a former CEO of the drug company Eli Lilly— announced in May that the Food and Drug Administration would institute an expedited drug-review process for the drugs in question. But it's still unclear how much time these reviews will take.

"If [the Bush administration] were operating in good faith, they would try to strengthen the [World Health Organization] process and engage in technical discussions with [the World Health Organization] on developing the combinations we so desperately need, like pediatric formulations," says Rachel Cohen, U.S. director of Doctors

Without Borders' Campaign for Essential Medicines. Instead, she says, they're seeking "to deny that these drugs meet international standards, because they don't want to set a precedent of using U.S. government money to finance medicines that are still on patent in the U.S." In addition, the U.S. trade representative's office is negotiating trade deals with poor countries that would impede them from quickly dispensing generic AIDS drugs.

There's one other step Bush could take if he was serious about fighting AIDS in Africa: Press for debt relief. Even Africa's creditors agree that debtor governments spend more money on hospitals and schools when offered debt cancellation: An International Monetary Fund fact sheet issued in April about 27 countries that have received partial debt relief reports that they "have increased markedly their expenditures on health, education and other social services."

In the case of Iraq, Bush has dispatched former Secretary of State James Baker as a special envoy on debt, and Baker is negotiating with foreign governments to waive 90 percent of Iraq's debt. But Bush has not even implemented the provision in his own AIDS law that would provide partial debt relief to African nations.

And so the situation remains bleak for AIDS workers in Africa, where an estimated 25 million people—out of a total of 38 million worldwide—are infected with HIV. Dr. Peter Mugyenyi was prominently seated next to first lady Laura Bush at last year's State of the Union address to applaud the president's stunning $15 billion announcement. Mugyenyi is now using a PEPFAR grant to the Joint Clinical Research Center of Uganda to provide free treatment to HIV-positive AIDS orphans. "We are very happy that we have sufficient money to be able to treat all of these kids without having to choose among them," says Mugyenyi.

But, as in the other PEPFAR countries, the vast majority of people in immediate need of AIDS drugs will go untreated. In Uganda, 150,000 to 200,000 people will not have access to the medicine they need, Mugyenyi says. "The expectation is very high that the drugs are coming," he notes carefully, "and we are hopeful that we are not going to disappoint them when they eventually find out that the drugs are not enough to go around."

Fatal Inaction

By Joshua Kurlantzick
The Washington Monthly, July/August 2006

Ndirande, Malawi, is one of the poorest neighborhoods in one of the poorest nations in the world. At a local health clinic, anxious mothers in brightly colored body wraps and head scarves shove their children's health records at the admissions counter. Inside, another 80 women wait for blood tests in a hot, tiny, windowless room, their babies suckling weakly at their breasts. Several babies lie unconscious or shaking on the ground. Others are so thin that their skeletal structures are plainly visible.

Twenty-three year old Margaret cradles her 11-month-old son in her arms. When he contracted malaria last week, she gave him Fansidar, a commonly prescribed antimalarial drug here. "He's not getting better," she says. Her voice cracks. Next to her, 25-year-old Innocent, a tall woman with long, wiry hair, has bundled her one-year-old in a heavy sweater to quell the chills that shake his small body. He's had malaria twice in the past two months, and also took Fansidar, with little effect. A physician's assistant moves from mother to mother, distributing pills that he knows are essentially' worthless. Most of the children in this room have had malaria before, and most will get it again: An African child dies of malaria nearly every 30 seconds.

Stories about Africa frequently hew to a familiar script: narratives of intractable tragedies ignored by the world with no feasible solutions in sight. This isn't one of those stories. Roger Bate, a malaria-policy expert at the American Enterprise Institute, calls malaria probably the most obviously preventable serious disease in Africa. Although the parasite has grown resistant to drugs that once tamed the disease—including the Fansidar distributed in the Ndirande clinic—it's easily treatable with a powerful drug called artemisinin. Nor has malaria escaped political attention. In 1998, Roll Back Malaria (an alliance of international organizations, including the World Bank and the United Nations) launched a campaign to halve global malaria deaths by 2010. Last year, President Bush called for a "broad, aggressive campaign" to cut malaria deaths in Africa by half an effort which, he declared, "our nation is prepared to lead."

Yet leadership has been noticeably absent from Washington's main aid-givers: the United States Agency for International Development and the World Bank. Both agencies have questioned artemisinin's effectiveness in the past, and squandered large portions of their malaria budgets. Meanwhile, malaria death rates have not decreased. Although some thoughtful conservatives like Sen. Sam Brownback have pushed USAID hard to address this entirely solvable problem, other conservatives have diverted reform energies by turning the issue into a partisan debate about environmental regulations. And the malaria crisis has received little tangible attention from the man who promised that "aggressive campaign" to fight it. After the president reaped considerable public praise for his declaration of support for Africa, he's shown less inclination to actually deliver the help that he promised.

ACT Up

Not that long ago, developed countries viscerally understood the connection between malaria and their own national health. Until the mid-20th century, the disease was a scourge of nearly every continent. The parasite, which travels from mosquitoes to humans,

---

Malaria, unlike HIV, lacks a vocal or wealthy Western constituency to push for the production of new drugs.

---

then through human blood to the liver, triggers fevers, nausea, and sometimes, deadly comas. Tellingly, major advances in treatment have often been spurred by economic ambitions. Malaria-control efforts were seen as crucial to the development of the American South, and became a linchpin of FDR's Tennessee Valley Authority Project, leading to the almost total eradication of the disease here by the late 1940s. But the effective disappearance of the disease from the developed world means that malaria, unlike HIV, lacks a vocal or wealthy Western constituency to push for the production of new drugs.

For a while, no new treatments were needed. Beginning in the 1950s, chloroquine halted malaria's march in Africa and Asia. But by the 1980s, the parasite had become resistant to the drug on both continents. The World Health Organization (WHO) termed chloroquine "useless"; other cheap drugs like Fansidar also lost their effectiveness. Now, at least 300 million cases of malaria occur annually. Ninety percent of the resulting deaths occur in Africa where the climate is particularly hospitable to mosquitoes. Severe epidemics are becoming common (almost half of Burundi's population of 6.5 million contracted malaria in 2001), and the number of children killed by the disease is rising. Malaria paralyzes economies too: recurring bouts keep children from school and adults from work. The disease is estimated to cost Africa as much as $12 billion in lost gross domestic product each year.

In the 1980s, a British researcher named Nick White helped develop the drug artemisinin, derived from a wormwood plant grown in southern China. White found that when artemisinin is combined with other drugs to form artemisinin-based combination therapy, or ACT, it cleared malaria from the blood in 90 percent of the cases. Clinics on the Thai-Burmese border were among the first in the world to use this remedy. In 2000, I visited one such clinic amid a thick, scrubby forest. Though the woods teemed with mosquitoes, only two women lay in the hut with their feverish children; as they played with their babies, they seemed convinced the kids would get better. They were right. By the end of the day, the children were running around the hut, and by nightfall, their mothers were able to take them home.

Using drugs manufactured in China and India, other Asian nations imitated White's success. Vietnam used ACT to slash infection rates by more than 97 percent in the 1990s. In 1999, prominent infectious disease specialists penned an article in the prestigious journal, *The Lancet*, calling for a rapid rollout of artemisinins in Africa. The following year, South Africa introduced an ACT called Coartem, manufactured by the Swiss pharmaceutical giant Novartis. Twelve months later, the number of cases in the South African province of KwaZulu Natal had plunged by almost 80 percent. In 2001 the World Health Organization recommended that all countries where malaria is resistant to older drugs should switch to ACT.

Most African nations accept that ACT should be their primary weapon in the war on malaria. At the central hospital in Lilongwe, Malawi's capital, Dr. Peter Kazembe's office is crammed with malaria studies and antiquated laptops that run malaria control models; his window overlooks a courtyard where young mothers wait anxiously for news of their sick children. (Virtually the entire population of Malawi is vulnerable to the disease.) As a pediatrician and longtime member of a government advisory committee on malaria control, Kazembe understands ACT's benefits. But Malawi, like most African countries, hasn't adopted ACT, partly because of the expense of the drugs. Kazembe considers his predicament: He knows exactly how to treat his patients, but he still can't help them. He laughs wryly, then excuses himself to leave for a funeral. "We spend so much time going to these things," he says.

Saving Lives vs. the Redskins

The cost of providing ACTs for the world's malaria sufferers is negligible by the standards of the rich world. For once, big pharma isn't the villain here. Novartis, which controls most of the ACT market, is willing to produce Coartem at cost. However, it won't boost production without guaranteed orders, according to people familiar with its operations. Until recently, donors couldn't purchase generics instead because, according to Médecins Sans Frontières, WHO has been slow to grant ACT produced in places like India the necessary pre-qualification status; under pressure, the WHO has started to step up pre-qualification. Without an increased supply, the price of artemisinin drugs is unlikely to fall. At the moment, the drugs run to about $2.50 per treatment, more than 20 times the cost of chloroquine, and well out of reach of the villagers in Malawi, for instance, where the average income is about 50 cents per day.

In 2004, the Institute of Medicine, a U.S. government scientific advisory body, proposed a global ACT subsidy to remedy this problem. The plan would require donor countries and multinational agencies to reserve up to $500 million to buy ACTs from companies like Novartis. (By comparison, $500 million is less than half the value of the Washington Redskins.) That way, Novartis and others could boost production knowing that orders were certain. The Institute noted that the subsidy would make ACTs available to all malaria sufferers for the same price as chloroquine—about 10 cents per treatment—and would actually stem future demand for anti-malarials: Unlike HIV treatments, which require long-term prescriptions of complicated antiretroviral drugs, ACT act rapidly and don't have to be taken indefinitely.

Dr. Francisco Saute is the deputy director of malaria control in Mozambique, which has one of Africa's highest malaria death rates. (One in every hundred Mozambican children dies from the disease.) A short man with a round face and a pug nose, Saute, who trained at elite institutions in Spain and Britain, shifts rapidly from English to Portuguese to Spanish. His cell phones trill constantly; he sweats rivulets out the front of his open-necked shirt. As he rushes between ten-minute meetings in the bowels of Mozambique's dilapidated, water-stained health ministry, he emits a stream of complaints. Some international health agencies, pressured by well-meaning activists, are pushing Mozambique to change its entire malaria infrastructure and buy artemisinins now—but won't provide the money to make the drugs affordable, he says. Mozambique did try to adopt ACT in 2004, with disastrous results when a surge in demand for Novartis caused a global shortage. One infectious disease doctor told me that some rural parts of Mozambique now have no malaria medications at all. "The international community pushed them to go to artemisinins, but with no way to pay for it," he says. Ramanan Laxminarayan, a malaria expert at the nonprofit Resources for the Future, believes that this situation could rapidly be solved if the United States threw its weight behind the subsidy. "African countries try to do what USAID wants them to do," he says. "It wouldn't take much time to get up and running once there is political will."

Africans Can Tell Time, Too

USAID was devised in 1961 as a tool in the Cold War. When that conflict ended, the agency faced fierce challenges to its relevance from conservative firebrands like Sen. Jesse Helms. Because of this pressure, in the 1990s, USAID's budget was slashed repeatedly and so was its staff—37 percent of the agency's staffers left or were not replaced. As a result, according to a report by AEI's Roger Bate, USAID became "largely a contracting organization." But by relying on American contractors to fulfill many of its mandates, USAID became far less accountable—as evidenced by its troubled malaria program.

USAID's malaria budget increased from $22 million in 1998 to $90 million by 2005. Last year, members of Congress held hearings to determine what that money had produced. The results weren't pretty. After interrogations from Sen. Tom Coburn and others, it emerged that in fiscal year 2004, USAID spent just 5 percent of its malaria budget on antimalarial drugs. The rest of the budget went to various "technical assistance" projects (such as a $65 million program for "social marketing" of mosquito nets to impoverished Africans), as well as salaries of U.S. consultants, travel expenses, training, and other services provided by American contractors. "We spent most of our money telling people how to use the cheap and effective tools to fight malaria," said Coburn at another hearing this January, "and very little money actually providing them those tools and very little money actually saving lives." Coburn has also questioned why the U.S. sinks its malaria cash into USAID, instead of supporting the Global Fund to Fight AIDS, Tuberculosis and Malaria, the major international organization that finances the purchase of malaria drugs. Bate concludes that most of USAID's malaria funds "either never left the United States . . . or funded the employment of U.S. citizens." Former USAID head Andrew Natsios admitted in 2003 that the organization has relied on contractors, but lacks the resources to oversee them: "We don't have enough officers to do the work," he told *Government Executive* magazine.

According to USAID's own internal reporting, as much as 80 percent of its total budget goes to American goods and American contractors. Disturbingly, it's almost impossible to know whether these

HOW USAID SPENDS ITS MALARIA MONEY

Total malaria budget for 2004: $80 million

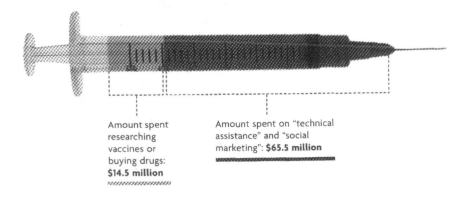

Amount spent researching vaccines or buying drugs: **$14.5 million**

Amount spent on "technical assistance" and "social marketing": **$65.5 million**

contractors provide value for money, as the agency is notoriously intransigent when it comes to evaluating its effectiveness. In 2000, economist Ruben Berrios found that USAID's bidding procedures were woefully uncompetitive, relying heavily on a small pool of contractors. The agency is also generally reluctant to release information on its work (dealing with the Pentagon is far easier). Bate points out that contractors have little incentive to actually solve the problems they're supposed to address, as successful advice would ultimately render them jobless.

But although USAID's inept response to malaria can partly be blamed on these institutional defects, even more troubling is the agency's apparent ambivalence towards ACT. Internal documents obtained by *The Washington Monthly* suggest that well after leading malaria experts recommended the benefits of ACT in *The Lancet*, USAID was still privately discouraging their use. "Let's not argue for . . . artemisinin therapy right now," reads a message from a 2001 email exchange between two of the agency's malaria specialists. Another message from 2003 suggests that the treatment should still be seriously debated—two years after the World Health Organization recommended a switch to artemisinins for countries where resistance had developed to older drugs. A 2004 *Lancet* article by 13 malaria specialists noted that countries that sought to switch to ACT were "forcefully pressured out of it" by the U.S. The resulting outcry forced USAID to declare support for ACT. In a meeting at USAID, agency disease experts told me that the organization had initially harbored concerns that countries would switch to ACT too quickly, before necessary infrastructure was in place. However, they said they recognized the importance of the powerful new treatment.

Some critics believe USAID had shunned artemisinin because of deep-seated doubts that Africans can handle complex treatments. In 2001, Natsios told a House committee hearing on HIV/AIDS that Africans "do not know what watches and clocks are." (Studies have shown that African patients correctly follow HIV drug regimens, which are more complicated than artemisinin combinations.) And although USAID commissioned the Institute of Medicine study that proposed subsidizing ACT, it has shown little inclination to support the plan. When I asked Peter Bloland of the Centers for Disease Control whether he'd seen the political will from Washington to push for the subsidy, he answered simply, "no."

Green Herring

Oddly, malaria has become something of a conservative *cause cele-bre* in recent years. Sen. Brownback has become a dedicated advocate for combating the disease. At congressional hearings, he and fellow Republican Sen. Coburn display an impressive knowledge of the crisis and the deficiencies of USAID's response. However, apart from a few such thoughtful exceptions, conservative energies have mostly been focused on another supposed solution: the insecticide DDT.

DDT, which helps kill malarial mosquitoes, was sprayed in America to eradicate malaria. But Rachel Carson's vivid portrayal of the horrors wrought by the chemical in her seminal book *Silent Spring* caused DDT to be banned in 1972, and helped launch the modern environmental movement. For some conservatives, malaria policy has now become an unlikely tool in the anti-environmentalist backlash. *The Weekly Standard*, The *Wall Street Journal* editorial page, and *National Review* have dedicated more than 10 editorials in recent years touting the benefits of DDT (although some conservatives like Bate, Brownback, and Coburn do advocate both DDT and ACT). At malaria hearings for the Senate Foreign Relations committee, Republican members have repeatedly asked why the United States doesn't promote DDT in malaria-stricken nations.

This preoccupation with DDT, however, is largely a distraction. Environmental leaders now agree that the pesticide should be used to combat malaria; few nations in Africa ban it; and USAID has agreed to spray DDT in countries like Ethiopia and Mozambique.

> For some conservatives, malaria policy has now become an unlikely tool in the anti-environmentalist backlash.

What's more, DDT is no silver bullet. Malaria experts agree that it reduces transmission, but emphasize that it must be combined with other interventions, including ACT. The furor over DDT has undoubtedly hampered efforts to provide better access to antimalarial drugs. When another malaria expert met with Senate staffers to discuss malaria in 2004 and 2005, they badgered him about DDT, "I tried to explain the reality," he says, "and people in the U.S. say 'That's not what I was told.'" "DDT has become a fetish," adds Allan Schapira of WHO. "You have people advocating DDT as if it's the only insecticide that works against malaria, as if DDT would solve all problems, which is obviously absolutely unrealistic."

Ultimately, despite the efforts of lawmakers like Brownback, meaningful action on malaria needs White House support. President Bush has certainly been generous with his rhetoric. Last year, he pledged $1.2 billion to the cause, challenging the world to move past "empty symbolism and discredited policies." However, Rep. Tom Lantos pointed out that for the first year, this sum didn't actually include any new money—it simply reallocated previously budgeted funds.

Stiffed by the World Bank

American inaction on ACT has fed a deeper malaise among both international and private institutions and private institutions that deal with malaria—and which tend to be heavily influenced by U.S. policy and funding. Last year, the Global Fund to Fight AIDS,

Tuberculosis and Malaria found itself $300 million short of the money it had planned to spend on drugs. President Bush had only requested $200 million for the Global Fund, less than half of what Congress had provided the previous year. But perhaps the most alarming example is the World Bank, which, according to a report in *The Lancet* this year, has failed to fulfill a 2000 promise to boost funding for malaria control. Instead, *The Lancet* found that the Bank funded obsolete drugs, downsized its malaria staff, and faked its financial accounts, possibly to mask mistakes. "No commercial high-street bank could keep such imprecise accounts for its clients, without running a serious risk of civil or criminal illegality," *The Lancet* concluded.

Some of the few hopeful signs are emerging from the private sector. In May 2005, the Bill & Melinda Gates Foundation pledged $35 million to a comprehensive anti-malaria pilot project in Zambia. The project combines all the possible antimalarial weapon—insecticides, bed nets, and ACT. The foundation also appears willing to fund a study to consider exactly how to deliver the global ACT subsidy; several major donor agencies including UNICEF and WHO are discussing how to make the subsidy work. Stung by congressional criticism, USAID also vowed in January to mend its ways (this year it intends to spend half of its malaria budget on drugs, nets and spraying). It has also said that it is rebuilding its staff to become less reliant on contractors. Whether these initiatives will bear fruit, or simply go the way of numerous other lofty goals, remains to be seen.

At Ndirande, a new crowd of children and mothers sits on the floor outside the doctor's office. The room echoes with the wails of skeletal babies. More worrisomely, some of the children are eerily silent. Meria cradles her baby daughter, who's been coughing up blood and vomiting repeatedly. Next to her, Agnes, a 46-year-old with a heavily-creased face who wears a headscarf decorated with brightly-colored mangoes, stares at her three-year-old son. He's not moving at all. "That boy has had malaria every month, and today he's having the same symptoms as before," Agnes says. "I'm worried he'll have this problem every month, forever.

APPENDIX

Bipartisan Group of Senators Introduce the African Health Capacity Investment Act of 2006

DURBIN.SENATE.GOV, AUGUST 3, 2006

A bipartisan group of Senators today introduced the African Health Capacity Investment Act of 2006, S.3775, a comprehensive bill to help sub-Saharan African nations confront the alarming shortage of health workers; thirteen countries on the continent have fewer than 5 physicians per 100,000 people. The United States has 549 physicians per 100,000 people.

Senators Dick Durbin (D-IL), Norm Coleman (R-MN), Russ Feingold (D-WI) and Mike DeWine (R-OH) called the lack of health care workers and capacity in many African nations a "critical obstacle" in the world's fight against HIV/AIDS and a potential outbreak of Avian Flu and in promoting economic development and growth.

"With 11 percent of the world's population, 25 percent of the global disease burden and nearly half of the world's deaths from infectious diseases, sub-Saharan Africa has only 3 percent of the world's health workers." Senator Durbin said. "Personnel shortages are a global problem, but nowhere are these shortages more extreme, the infrastructure more limited and the health challenges graver than in sub-Saharan Africa, the epicenter of the HIV/AIDS pandemic. We will not win the war against AIDS or any other health challenge without finding solutions to this crisis," Durbin said.

"I am very proud to join my colleagues in introducing this bill as it is critical for bolstering our efforts to combat HIV/AIDS and other diseases in Africa," said Senator Coleman. "The lack of health care capacity in Africa imposes major constraints on the long term effectiveness of programs fighting HIV/AIDS and other diseases. For this reason, any forward-looking, comprehensive strategy to fight these terrible diseases must include elements that build African health care capacity."

"The massive shortage of healthcare workers may be the most critical issue facing health care systems in Africa, contributing to millions of preventable deaths each year," Senator Feingold said. "I am proud of the leadership role the United States has taken in addressing HIV/AIDS, malaria, tuberculosis, and other global health crises. However, the resources we have invested in Africa will ultimately be fruitless unless we establish an infrastructure to ensure their effectiveness in the long-term."

"I am proud to join my colleagues in supporting this worthy bill that will help millions of people in Africa get the basic health services they need. A coordinated strategy for healthcare workers would ultimately help combat the HIV/AIDS epidemic by increasing treatment and education about the disease. This, coordinated with infrastructure improvements, will also give much needed doctors and nurses access to more patients," said Senator DeWine. "In addition, these measures will help these developing nations to support economic growth and create jobs for their citizens."

The African Health Capacity Investment Act of 2006 seeks to help sub-Saharan African countries strengthen the capabilities of their health systems by:

Improving dangerous and sub-standard working conditions; Helping train, recruit, and retain doctors, nurses, and paraprofessionals; Developing better management and public health training; and Improving productivity and workforce distribution.

The bill also seeks to promote enhanced coordination of U.S. foreign assistance and requires the President to develop a coordinated strategy to promote health care capacity in Africa.

From Remarks by the President on the G8 Summit

PRESIDENT GEORGE W. BUSH
WWW.WHITEHOUSE.GOV, JUNE 30, 2005

. . . Today, in Africa, the United States is engaged as never before. We're seeing great progress, and great needs remain. So this morning, I announced three additional initiatives to help Africans address urgent challenges. Across the continent, there is a deep need for the empowerment of women, and that begins with education. Educated young women have lower rates of HIV/AIDS, healthier families, and higher rates of education for their own children. Yet only half of the children complete primary education in Africa.

Together with African leaders, we must work for the education of every African child. And to move closer to that goal, today, I proposed a double funding for America's African Education Initiative. (Applause.) In the next four years, we should provide $400 million to train half-a-million teachers, and provided scholarships for 300,000 young people, mostly girls. (Applause.) We hope other nations will join us. We must give more girls in Africa a real chance to avoid exploitation and to chart their own future.

Another important aspect of empowerment and the fight against AIDS is the legal protection of women and girls against sexual violence and abuse. (Applause.) Many African nations have already taken steps to improve legal rights for women. South Africa, for example, has an innovative model to fight rape and domestic violence: special units in hospitals where victims can report crime and receive counseling and care, and special judges and prosecutors and police units to ensure that criminals are punished.

Today, I announce a new effort to spread this approach more broadly on the continent. I ask Congress to provide $55 million over three years to promote women's justice and empowerment in four African nations, nations that can stand as examples of reform for others. I'll urge other G8 nations to join us in protecting the lives and the rights of women in Africa.

African health officials have also told us of their continuing battle with malaria, which in some countries can cause more death than AIDS. Approximately 1 million last year alone died on the African continent because of malaria. And in the overwhelming majority of cases, the victims are less than five years old, their lives suddenly ended by nothing more than a mosquito bite. The toll of malaria is even more tragic because the disease, itself, is highly treatable and preventable. Yet this is also our opportunity, because we know that large-scale action can defeat this disease in whole regions. And the world must take action. (Applause.)

Next week at the G8, I will urge developed countries and private foundations to join in a broad, aggressive campaign to cut the mortality rate for malaria across Africa in half. And our nation is prepared to lead. (Applause.) Next year, we will take comprehensive action in three countries—Tanzania, Uganda and Angola—to provide indoor spraying, long-lasting insecticide-treated nets, and effective new combination drugs to treat malaria. In addition, the Gates Foundation of Seattle is supporting a major effort to control malaria in Zambia. We've had a long tradition of public-private action. I'm grateful to have this strong partner in a good cause.

America will bring this anti-malaria effort to at least four more highly endemic African countries in 2007, and at least to five more in 2008. In the next five years, with the approval of Congress, we'll spend more than $1.2 billion on this campaign. (Applause.)

An effort on this scale must be phased in, to avoid shortages of supplies. Yet we intend this effort to eventually cover more than 175 million people in 15 or more nations. We want to reduce malaria mortality in target countries by half, and save hundreds of thousands of lives.

I urge other wealthy nations and foundations to participate and expand this initiative to additional countries where the need is pressing. Together, we can live this threat and defeat this fear across the African continent. . . .

Delivered at the Smithsonian Institution's Freer Gallery of Art in Washington, D.C., June 30, 2005.

BIBLIOGRAPHY

Books

African Health Sciences Congress. *24th African Health Sciences Congress: Challenges and Strategies in Combating Health Problems in Africa, Towards Development Efforts: African Union Conference Centre, Addis Ababa, Ethiopia, Sept. 2–Oct. 2, 2003: Congress Abstracts /Organized by the Ethiopian Health & Nutrition Research Institute (EHNRI) in Collaboration with African Union (AU), African Forum for Health Sciences (AFHES), and World Health Organization (WHO)*. Addis Ababa, Ethiopia: EHNRI: AU: AFHES: WHO, 2003.

Belsey, Mark A. *AIDS and the Family: Policy Options for a Crisis in Family Capital*. New York: United Nations, Department of Economic and Social Affairs, 2005.

Blackden, C. Mark, and Quentin Wodon, eds. *Gender, Time Use, and Poverty in Sub-Saharan Africa*. Washington, D.C.: World Bank, 2006.

Center for Reproductive Law and Policy. *Women of the World: Laws and Policies Affecting Their Reproductive Lives: Anglophone Africa, Progress Report 2001*. 1st ed. New York, NY: Center for Reproductive Law and Policy, 2001.

Chirimuuta, Richard C. (Richard Chidau). *AIDS, Africa, and Racism*. London: Free Association Books, 1989.

Djamba, Yanyi K., ed. *Sexual Behavior of Adolescents in Contemporary Sub-Saharan Africa*. Lewiston, N.Y.: Edwin Mellen Press, 2004.

Ernst, Waltraud, ed. *Plural Medicine, Tradition and Modernity, 1800–2000*. New York: Routledge, 2002.

Ewbank, Douglas C., and James N. Gribble, eds. *Effects of Health Programs on Child Mortality in Sub-Saharan Africa; Working Group on the Effects of Child Survival and General Health Programs on Mortality, Panel on the Population Dynamics of Sub-Saharan Africa, Committee on Population, Commission on Behavioral and Social Sciences and Education, National Research Council*. Washington, D.C.: National Academy Press, 1993.

Guest, Emma. *Children of AIDS: Africa's Orphan Crisis*. Sterling, Va.: Pluto Press; Pietermaritzburg, South Africa: University of Natal Press, 2001.

Howard, W. Stephen, and Arvind Singhal. *The Children of Africa Confront AIDS: From Vulnerability to Possibility*. Athens: Ohio University Press, 2003.

Howson, Christopher P., ed. *In Her Lifetime: Female Morbidity and Mortality in Sub-Saharan Africa / Committee to Study Female Morbidity and Mortality in Sub-Saharan Africa, Board on International Health, Institute of Medicine*. Washington, D.C.: National Academy Press, 1996.

Jackson, Helen. *AIDS Africa: Continent in Crisis*. Harare, Zimbabwe: SAfAIDS, 2002.

Jamison, Dean T. *Disease and Mortality in Sub-Saharan Africa*. 2nd ed. Washington, D.C.: World Bank, 2006.

Kalipeni, Ezekiel, and Philip Thiuri. *Issues and Perspectives on Health Care in Contemporary Sub-Saharan Africa.* Lewiston, N.Y.: Edwin Mellen Press, 1997.

Keller, Edmond J., and Donald Rothchild eds. *Africa-US Relations: Strategic Encounters.* Boulder, Colo.: Lynne Rienner, 2006.

Kelly, M. J. *The Encounter Between HIV/AIDS and Education.* Harare, Zimbabwe: UNESCO Sub-Regional Office for Southern Africa, 2000.

Kempe, Ronald Hope, Sr., ed. *AIDS and Development in Africa: A Social Science Perspective.* New York: Haworth Press, 1999.

Koop, C. Everett, Clarence E. Pearson, and M. Roy Schwarz. *Critical Issues in Global Health.* 1st ed. San Francisco: Jossey-Bass, 2002.

Mati, J. K. G. *AIDS, Women and Children in Africa: The Impact of AIDS on Reproductive Health.* Nairobi, Kenya: IRHTR, 1997.

Morisky, Donald E. *Overcoming AIDS: Lessons Learned from Uganda.* Greenwich, Conn.: IAP-Information Age Pub., 2006.

Mwabu, Germano M. *Poverty and Malaria in Africa: A Research and Policy Agenda.* Nairobi, Kenya: African Economic Research Consortium, 2002.

———. *Health and Growth in Africa.* Nairobi, Kenya: Kenya Institute for Public Policy Research and Analysis, 2004.

Ngom, Pierre. *Demographic Surveillance and Health Equity in Sub-Saharan Africa: Past and Present Efforts.* Nairobi, Kenya: African Population & Health Research Center, 2001.

———. *Fertility Decline in Francophone Sub-Saharan Africa, 1980–2010.* Nairobi, Kenya: African Population & Health Research Center, 2002.

Nordberg, Erik, ed. *Communicable Diseases: A Manual for Health Workers in Sub-Saharan Africa.* 3rd ed. Nairobi, Kenya: African Medical and Research Foundation, 1999.

O'Manique, Colleen. *Neoliberalism and AIDS Crisis in Sub-Saharan Africa: Globalization's Pandemic.* New York: Palgrave Macmillan, 2004.

Peters, David H., ed. *Health Expenditures, Services, and Outcomes in Africa: Basic Data and Cross-national Comparisons, 1990–1996.* Washington, D.C.: World Bank, 1999.

Subbarao, K. *Reaching Out to Africa's Orphans: A Framework for Public Action.* Washington, D.C.: World Bank, 2004.

Turshen, Meredeth. *Privatizing Health Services in Africa.* New Brunswick, N.J.: Rutgers University Press, 1999.

United States Congress, Committee on International Relations. *Subcommittee on Africa, Malaria and Tuberculosis in Africa: Hearing Before the Subcommittee on Africa of the Committee on International Relations, House of Representatives, One Hundred Eighth Congress, Second Session, September 14, 2004.* Washington, D.C.: U.S. G.P.O., 2004.

Vogel, Ronald J. *Financing Health Care in Sub-Saharan Africa.* Westport, Conn.: Greenwood Press, 1993.

Waite, Gloria Martha. *A History of Traditional Medicine and Health Care in Pre-colonial East-Central Africa.* Lewiston, N.Y.: E. Mellen Press, 1992.

World Bank. *Improving Health, Nutrition, and Population Outcomes in Sub-Saharan Africa: The Role of the World Bank.* Washington, D.C.: World Bank, 2005.

World Bank Group, Human Development, Africa Region. *Education and Health in Sub-Saharan Africa: A Review of Sector-wide Approaches.* Washington: World Bank, 2001.

Web Sites

Readers seeking additional information about global epidemics may wish to refer to the following Web sites, all of which were operational as of this writing.

African Business
www.africasia.com/africanbusiness/

This homepage for the magazine African Business provides archived articles, current issues, and information about economics in Africa.

Africare
www.africare.org/

This Web site describes the activities of the nonprofit organization that offers aid to Africa and describes ways that everyone can help.

Bill & Melinda Gates Foundation
www.gatesfoundation.org/default.htm

The site provides information about issues important to the foundation and supplies avenues of financial assistance, including details about the organization's Global Health Program.

Centers for Disease Control and Prevention (CDC)
www.cdc.gov/

This government agency is devoted to research into preventing and treating all types of health disorders.

The Global Fund to Fight AIDS, Tuberculosis and Malaria
www.theglobalfund.org/en/

This Web site of the nonprofit organization is dedicated to fighting these three potentially deadly diseases around the world.

Medilinks
medilinkz.org/HealthTopics/safehealthcare/safehealthcare.asp

This site offers general information about health care, with a special section on safe health care in Africa.

SULAIR: Africa South of the Sahara
www-sul.stanford.edu/africa/health.html

Stanford University maintains this site, with links to articles, databases, and Web sites concerning African studies.

United Nations Economic Commission for Africa
www.uneca.org/

This UN committee works to improve economic conditions and health care provisions throughout the continent.

The United States President's Emergency Plan for AIDS Relief
www.pepfar.gov/

This site lists the goals and accomplishes of President Bush's plan to fight AIDS throughout the world.

World Bank
www.worldbank.org/

Along with descriptions of this nongovernmental organization and its mission throughout the world, the site explains the goals and activities of its international programs, including the Africa Action Plan to improve quality of life and reduce poverty in the region.

UN AIDS
www.unaids.org/en/

The site provides information about the Joint United Nations Programme on HIV/AIDS, in which 10 UN organizations are working together to address the AIDS crisis throughout the world.

UN Millennium Development Goals
www.un.org/millenniumgoals/

Here, one can find a list of the 10 goals, to be reached by 2015, developed by the United Nations to help the world's poorest people.

World Health Organization
www.who.int/en/

This site supplies statistics, charts, pamphlets, and reports about the state of health throughout the world.

Additional Periodical Articles with Abstracts

More information about free trade and related subjects can be found in the following articles. Readers who require a more comprehensive selection are advised to consult *Business Abstracts, Humanities Abstracts, Readers' Guide Abstracts, Social Science Abstracts,* and other H.W. Wilson publications.

Malaria: Sub-Saharan Africa. *America,* v. 190 p3 May 10, 2004.

An unusual sort of indifference sets in when it comes to addressing so-called neglected diseases such as malaria, which actually kills more than 1 million people every year. Humanitarian health organizations such as Doctors Without Borders believe that cost considerations have restricted the wider use of artemisinin-based combination therapy (ACT), but there has also been a lack of political will on the part of international donor nations and governments in malaria-ravaged regions to switch to ACT. Moreover, with malaria almost entirely eliminated in wealthy countries, the for-profit pharmaceutical industry is undertaking hardly any research into treatment.

Origins of HIV: The Interrelationship between Nonhuman Primates and the Virus. Myrna E. Watanabe. *BioScience,* v. 54 pp810–14 September 2004.

The search for the origins of human immunodeficiency virus (HIV) has centered on the jungles of central Africa, where wild primates are endemic, Watanabe writes. By the mid-1980s, researchers had identified in captive, laboratory primates simian immunodeficiency virus (SIV), a virus similar to HIV. Bette Korber and colleagues then produced a seminal paper in the June 9, 2000, issue of *Science,* which stated that HIV-1, the predominant HIV virus, is most closely related to the chimpanzee SIV found in western equatorial Africa, and that transmission into humans probably occurred around 1930. In total, SIV has jumped into humans and caused disease at least 10 times.

Death in Africa: UNAIDS Workshop in Dakar, Senegal. Steven Englund. *Commonweal,* v. 126 pp8–9 August 13, 1999.

In June, UNAIDS organized a workshop in Dakar, Senegal, entitled "International Alliance for a Religious Response to AIDS in Africa" to address the persistent stigma attached to AIDS-HIV on the continent. Since the epidemic began, 83 percent of all AIDS deaths have occurred in sub-Saharan Africa, and in some regions perhaps as much as one-third of the population aged 15–49 is infected with the virus. Many infected people refuse what little care is available because of the shame associated with the disease, however. Moreover, although early and sustained prevention efforts would certainly reduce African HIV-infection rates, only 4 or 5 of the 35 or so governments in the region have publicly acknowledged the epidemic. The conference, attended mainly by individuals active in health care and religion, attempted to bring pressure on governments to enact public AIDS policies.

Why Do So Many Africans Get AIDS? Josie Glausiusz. *Discover*, v. 24 p12 June 2003.

According to four reports by Gisselquist and colleagues in the International Journal of STD & AIDS, heterosexual sex may not be the dominant transmission route for AIDS in Africa. Based on their analysis of 20 years of epidemiological research, the investigators concluded that most AIDS transmission in Africa is caused by unsafe injections, blood transfusions, and other medical procedures. Their data suggest that no more than 35 percent of HIV in adults is transmitted via sexual intercourse. Gisselquist says that medical researchers may have overemphasized sexual transmission of AIDS in Africa partly because condom-use campaigns fit with their concerns regarding overpopulation and because they are worried that Africans will lose faith in modern health care.

Africa's Custom-Made Cures. Martin Enserink. *Foreign Policy*, p84–5 January/February 2004.

Enserink discusses an article on the Ebola virus, written by Barry Hewlett and Richard Amola, that was published in the October 2003 issue of Emerging Infectious Diseases. In the article, Hewlett, an anthropologist at Washington State University, and Amola, a medical official at the Ugandan Ministry of Health, discussed the research they conducted on the cultural context of Ebola among a Ugandan ethnic group known as the Acholi. The researchers discovered that the Acholi—who believed that the illness was caused by bad spirits, perhaps as punishment for not respecting the gods—were combating the virus by using such sensible containment procedures as quarantine. This prompted Hewlett and Amola to conclude that traditional beliefs are not always an obstacle in containing epidemics.

Sub-Saharan Africa: At the Turning Point. Shanti R. Conly. *The Humanist*, v. 58 pp19–23 July/August 1998.

Sub-Saharan Africa is at a crucial turning point, Conly writes, in its attempts to introduce significant changes in government family-planning policies and general attitudes toward childbearing. Strong evidence of a fundamental change in views on childbearing could benefit the health of women and children, and some African governments are significantly improving reproductive-health services. An effective alliance between sub-Saharan Africa's governments, donor countries, and the private sector is necessary in order to meet the region's population-growth and reproductive-health challenges.

Clinton and Mandela Push for More Money, Determination to Fight Worldwide AIDS Epidemic. *Jet*, v. 102 pp54–6 July 29, 2002.

The writer discusses efforts by former U.S. president Bill Clinton and former South African president Nelson Mandela to persuade world leaders of the threat posed by AIDS to international peace and economic stability.

Clinton Makes Strong Appeal for U.S. Funds and Support for Africa. *Jet*, v. 97 pp4+ March 6, 2000.

President Clinton has promised to come to the rescue of the neglected and long-suffering continent of Africa. Speaking to the National Summit on Africa in the Washington Convention Center, Clinton, the first American president to visit Africa while in office, asserted that the United States should provide more support for disease control, debt relief, and conflict resolution in Africa. Almost 3,000 guests gathered for the Ford Foundation–financed, five-day conference, which is one of the largest volunteer crowds ever organized to promote an African cause. Summit sponsors hoped the black community could add momentum to the drive to support Africa.

AIDS in Africa. *The Nation*, v. 271 p4–5 August 7–14, 2000.

The increasing infection rates with AIDS gave the 13th International AIDS Conference in Durban, South Africa, a sense of heightened urgency. Although South African president Thabo Mbeki has been criticized for entertaining discredited theories on the disease, he is right to have discussed the substantially ignored role of the region's extreme poverty. Wealthy nations must take some basic steps to address sub-Saharan Africa's AIDS crisis, including the facilitating of the manufacture and sale of generic versions of AIDS drugs. Even if cheap drugs are available, the region will still need massive amounts of capital to build the kind of health care systems necessary for long-term drug therapy, however.

Living with AIDS. Gideon Mendel. *National Geographic*, v. 208 p66–73 September 2005.

In a special issue on Africa, Mendel writes that HIV/AIDS has become a fact of life and death in the rural Lusikisiki area of South Africa. In some ways, sufferers in this part of the Eastern Cape Province are more fortunate than most of the Africans battling the disease, with almost 800 people there receiving antiretroviral drugs in the past two years. The medication is administered by Siyaphila La, a joint initiative of the Nelson Mandela Foundation, Médicins Sans Frontières South Africa, and the local health department that is proving wrong the widely held notion that the three-pill drug therapy used in the West is too expensive and too complicated to use in impoverished African communities. The organization is also addressing the social stigma linked with HIV/AIDS by treating it as a manageable chronic illness. In a photo-essay, people in Lusikisiki relate how HIV/AIDS has changed their lives.

Medical Error: Consumer-driven Health Plans in South Africa. David Adler. *The New Republic*, v. 233 pp16–17 November 7, 2005.

Adler writes that the experience of South Africa should serve as a cautionary tale for proponents of health savings accounts. Many business leaders and conservative law makers in the United States are touting the ability of health savings accounts to fix the problems in U.S. health care. In South Africa, where the health system is not dissimilar to that in the United States, consumer-driven health care has attracted the young and healthy but isolated the old and infirm. Moreover, private health care costs there have increased, and there have been significant rises in plans' administrative costs. In addition, the number of South Africans lacking health insurance has continued to grow rapidly.

A Worldwide Gender Gap. Kati Marton. *Newsweek*, v. 143 p94 May 10, 2004.

In this special issue on women's health, Marton writes that women receive insufficient medical care in many societies, and they do not suffer the consequences of this situation alone. Healthy women are the basis of healthy families, which encourage healthy, prosperous societies. Although experience demonstrates that even small investments in women's health can pay substantial social dividends, few of those who could make these investments are doing so. The gender gap in health is particularly dramatic in the HIV/AIDS epidemic: In sub-Saharan Africa, women make up 60 percent of those with AIDS.

Bush Pushes South African in Fighting AIDS. Richard W. Stevenson. *The New York Times* (Late New York Edition) ppA1+, July 10, 2003.

Stevenson discusses President Bush's promised money to fight AIDS in South Africa, which has been slow to attack the disease. He urged President Thabo Mbeki to deal with the epidemic more forcefully.

Circumcision Studied in Africa as AIDS Preventive. Sharon LaFraniere. *The New York Times*, (Late New York Edition) ppA1+ April 28, 2006.

LaFraniere states that clinics all over Southern Africa are offering circumcisions in order to stem the rise of new HIV infections. Research found that the cells on the underside of the foreskin are prime targets of the HIV virus. Evidence suggests that circumcision may lower the risk of HIV infections by 30 percent.

Free AIDS Drugs in Africa Offer Dose of Life. Rachel L. Swarns. *The New York Times*, (Late New York Edition) ppA1 February 8, 2003.

According to Swarns, a vast majority of AIDS patients in South Africa die because they cannot afford the lifesaving medicines common in the West. But over the past two years, a number of private initiatives offering free or low-cost AIDS drugs have been started. One of the largest free programs is run by the relief agency Doctors Without Borders in Khayelitsha township near Cape Town. They provide free triple-therapy treatment to about 330 people and report remarkable results. This article profiles the Doctors Without Borders AIDS clinic in Khayelitsha.

Malaria Vaccine Proves Effective. Donald G. McNeil Jr. *The New York Times* p1 October 15, 2004.

McNeil shows that a vaccine produced by GlaxoSmithKline has been proven to be the most effective remedy in the fight against malaria so far. After extensive tests on children in Mozambique, researchers found that it may prevent the disease 30 percent of the time and tamed malaria in 58 percent of the cases. Malaria kills more than 1 million people every year, 700,000 of them children.

Push for New Tactics as War on Malaria Falters. Celia Dugger. *The New York Times*, (Late New York Edition) ppA1+ June 28, 2006.

Dugger states that paltry budgets, faulty strategies, and government mismanagement have hobbled efforts to combat malaria, which claims the lives of 800,000 African children each year. Despite increased funding for malaria eradication and control, little of it was spent on low-cost solutions like mosquito netting and mosquito repellent. Money was spent instead on high-priced consultants. Intense scrutiny, combined with a windfall of new financing is prompting new donors to devise new ways to stamp out the disease.

A Real-World AIDS Vaccine? Tina Rosenberg. *The New York Times Magazine*, pp15–16 January 14, 2007.

According to Rosenberg, scientific research findings indicate that circumcision helps to protect men from contracting the AIDS virus and may also protect their sexual partners. There is as yet no sign of a perfect AIDS vaccine being developed, but circumcision and the vaccine together might be sufficient to stop AIDS, provided that such interventions as behavior change, microbicides, fighting malaria, and treating genital herpes are also implemented. In the hands of traditional ritual circumcisers, the procedure has a high rate of infection and mishap, and it is therefore important to train these circumcisers and provide them with decent tools, as well as encouraging men to come to clinics.

What the World Needs Now Is DDT: Malaria Control. Tina Rosenberg. *The New York Times Magazine*, pp38–43 April 11, 2004.

Rosenberg writes that the United States frowns on the use of dichloro-diphenyl-tricholrethane (DDT) in developing nations, even though, if used carefully, it could significantly reduce the number of deaths caused by malaria. In South Africa, DDT is used to spray the inside walls of homes in infected regions once every 12 months, and it is also used for routine malaria control in a further five other countries. Nonetheless, the chemical has been outlawed in the United States since 1972, and its presence in the ecosystem, where it builds up to wipe out birds and fish, is symbolic of its risks. The continuance of DDT's deadly image in the West and the disproportionate weight that U.S. decisions carry globally are two of the reasons why DDT remains essentially unobtainable for most malarial countries.

Access for All? Joep M. A. Lange and Vallop Thaineua. *Science*, v. 304 p1875 June 25, 2004.

Addressing the HIV epidemic globally calls for an organized mechanism that recognizes basic economic realities, argue Lange and Thaineua. Although the prevalence of adult HIV infection in parts of sub-Saharan Africa represents an unprecedented scale of human suffering, provision of therapy there is inadequate because many of the hardest-hit countries in sub-Saharan Africa are failed states in which the public sector is unable to offer basic health services to the masses. Scaling-up treatment in resource-poor countries and minimizing the impact of HIV in developed nations will only succeed and prevail if robust insurance schemes have been established to provide sustainable financing of comprehensive health care for the masses.

AIDS and Africa: Still a Sad Story. Donald Kennedy. *Science*, v. 300 p1053 May 16, 2003.

President Bush's commitment of $15 billion to combat the AIDS epidemic in Africa is welcome news, but much remains to be done, Kennedy writes. Not all of the promised $15 billion is new money; about $5 billion is made up of previous annual commitments, and most of the allocation will be deferred to later years. In the countries affected, there are still many problems. In South Africa, for example, skepticism from the Mbeki government has hampered progress for the 5 million citizens who are infected.

Fighting Tropical Diseases. Peter J. Hotez and Jeffrey D. Sachs. *Science*, v. 311 p1521 March 17, 2006.

Hotez and Sachs write that the promise of a science-based policy approach to the fight against poverty, hunger, and disease is illustrated by a new effort to control several of the major killer infectious diseases. The initiative is prompted by recent analyses that indicate that the disease burden imposed by neglected tropical diseases has been underestimated and by the knowledge that chronic parasitic infections may increase an individual's risk of acquiring AIDS, tuberculosis, or malaria. The effort, which was planned by experts at a January meeting at the Karolinska Institute in Stockholm, Sweden, will initially focus on 10 countries that have pledged to have comprehensive scale-up plans to fight malaria and neglected tropical diseases ready by the end of April. Funding will be sought from the Global Fund to Fight AIDS, Tuberculosis, and Malaria, the World Bank, and other sources. A coordinated assault on tropical infections could become one of the most valuable projects in all of public health if successful.

Health Workers Scramble to Contain African Epidemic. Leslie Roberts. *Science*, v. 305 pp24–5 July 2, 2004.

Global health officials are preparing for the worst polio epidemic in years in western and central Africa, Roberts explains. In late 2003, the northern Nigerian state of Kano suspended vaccination activities over fears that the vaccine had been intentionally contaminated to cause infertility or AIDS in the largely Muslim population. Subsequently, Nigeria was hit by a polio epidemic, with 257 cases confirmed by June 22, and the virus spread to 10 polio-free countries, including conflict-ravaged Sudan. The situation is particularly worrisome because these cases are occurring in the so-called low season, when the transmission of poliovirus usually ebbs. David L. Heynmann, the WHO's representative for polio eradication, has announced that in response, the global polio eradication initiative hopes to carry out two huge coordinated immunization rounds in 22 African countries, beginning as early as October, with the aim of immunizing 74 million children at least twice, approximately one month apart.

HIV/AIDS Control in Sub-Saharan Africa: Discussion of Resource Needs for HIV/AIDS. Stefan Hanson, B. Schwartlander, and Neff Walker. *Science*, v. 294 no. 5542 p.521–3 October 19, 2001.

Although money and drugs are needed to control HIV/AIDS in sub-Saharan Africa, the writers claim there is a greater need for operational systems that can absorb funds and effectively convert them into care and prevention. Furthermore, although implementation of control strategies cannot depend entirely on government systems, it has to be carried out in close cooperation with them in order to achieve reasonable coverage. Smaller, nongovernmental agencies with a proven track record could be used to smooth operations, but, regardless of how aid plans are implemented, there must be simultaneous support for sector reforms and individual projects.

Malaria—a Shadow over Africa. Brian Greenwood and Louis H. Miller. *Science*, v. 298 pp121–2 October 4, 2002.

Greenwood and Miller propose that publication of the genomes of the malaria-causing parasite *Plasmodium falciparum* and its mosquito vector, *A. gambiae*, represents a major step forward in the search for new tools for controlling malaria. New, more effective, and inexpensive public health measure are required to achieve a reduction in severe disease and death from *P. falciparum* malaria in Africa. Combined deployment of drug treatment, vaccination, and vector control should be sufficient to stop malaria transmission, even in highly endemic areas of Africa. The complete genome sequences of *P. falciparum* and *A. gambiae* will be essential to this undertaking.

Will a Preemptive Strike Against Malaria Pay Off? Gretchen Vogel. *Science*, v. 310 pp1606–7 December 9, 2005.

According to Vogel, researchers are testing a bold new strategy aimed at protecting infants and children from malaria. The strategy, called intermittent preventative treatment (IPT), involves routinely giving anti-malaria drugs to infants regardless of whether they are infected with malaria parasites. The WHO already recommends that all pregnant women in malaria-affected regions receive IPT. Early trials of IPT in infants in Tanzania had remarkable results, but further studies have not been as positive. The biggest concern is that the strategy could backfire by increasing the malaria parasite's drug resistance. A sidebar highlights new evidence that the parasite has developed resistance to artemisin-based drugs.

AIDS Drugs for Africa. Carol Ezzell. *Scientific American*, v. 283 pp98–103 November 2000.

Ezzell shows that there are many factors preventing AIDS treatments from reaching Africa. Mother-to-child transmission of HIV is one of the driving forces behind the AIDS pandemic in Africa, but the antiretroviral drug regimens for preventing this transmission are virtually unavailable. The high cost of antiretroviral drugs is critically important, but many argue that there are other impediments, including poverty, globalization, and lack of health care infrastructure. Furthermore, there are the costs of the testing necessary to measure the success of the drugs in individual patients and to monitor the emergence of resistant virus. Also, few leaders of sub-Saharan African countries have supported the use of antiretroviral drugs

The Neglected Tropical Diseases. Jeffrey D. Sachs. *Scientific American*, v. 296 p33A January 2007.

A relatively modest amount of money could control neglected tropical diseases (NTDs) that afflict millions of poor people worldwide, Sachs states. Thirteen NTDs—7 helminth worm infections, 3 protozoan infections, and 3 bacterial infections—maim and kill as many people as AIDS, tuberculosis, and malaria but are less well-known because they only affect poor people in the tropics. There are powerful, low-cost, easily administered preventive or curative interventions for 9 of these diseases, and a comprehensive, Africa-wide strategy to control malaria and NTDs together would probably cost no more than $3 billion a year, which is the equivalent of just two days of spending by the Pentagon. According to Sachs, it is time for governments to join the efforts of drug companies and others in fighting NTDs.

Aids in South Africa: An Historical Perspective. Howard Phillips. *Society*, v. 40 4 pp72–6 May/June 2003.

Phillips explains that there has been a relative failure by historians of South Africa to make prior epidemic experiences part of the mainstream narrative of the nation's history. The writer attempts to remedy this omission and suggests that if AIDS in South Africa is put into the comparative perspective of the country's epidemic history, people's ability to understand it will be expanded considerably.

Malaria in Africa Today. Erika Reinhardt. *UN Chronicle*, v. 41 p. 72 March/May 2004.

According to the UN, Malaria kills one child every 30 seconds and over 1 million people each year in Africa. The Africa Malaria Report of 2003 reports that the disease continues to take its toll on extremely young children, chiefly those under the age of five, and pregnant women south of the Sahara. New analyses confirm that malaria is the main cause of at least 20 percent of all deaths of young children in the area. In endemic countries, up to one-third of all clinic visits and at least 25 percent of all hospital admissions are due to malaria. The Summit on Roll Back Malaria, which took place in Abuja, Nigeria, in 2002, endorsed some fairly inexpensive but effective control interventions already available, including insecticide-treated nets (ITNs) that have proven to be very effective in cutting mortality in young children. The writer discusses the efficacy of ITNs and other treatment options.

Where a Child Dies Each Minute: Vaccination of Children Against Measles in Sub-Saharan Africa. Phyllis A. Cuttino. *UN Chronicle*, v. 39 p26 June/August 2002.

According to Cuttino, although measles death can be prevented with a simple and inexpensive vaccine, 450,000 children die from the disease annually in Africa. As a result, the Measles Initiative has been established, with the long-term aim of vaccinating around 200 million children at risk throughout Africa. Through supplemental and follow-up campaigns in more than 30 sub-Sarahan nations, approximately 1.2 million deaths will be prevented, bringing measles fatalities in the region to almost nothing by 2005. The Measles Initiative is a U.S.-based partnership that combines the technical expertise, experience, and strength of the UN Foundation, the American Red Cross, the Centers for Disease Control and Prevention, UNICEF, and the World Health Organization.

WHO Report 2005: TB Linked to HIV at Alarming Levels in Africa. Erika Reinhardt. *UN Chronicle*, v. 42 pp17–19 June/August 2005.

In Africa, an increasing number of cases of tuberculosis (TB) are linked to HIV, according to the World Health Organization (WHO). The organization's WHO Report 2005, Global Tuberculosis Control: Surveillance, Planning, Financing, issued on March 24 to coincide with World TB Day, finds that the prevalence of TB has fallen worldwide by over 20 percent since 1990 and that incidence rates are falling or stable in all regions apart from Africa. It notes that in Africa, however, TB rates have tripled since 1990, in countries with high HIV prevalence and continue to increase at 3 to 4 percent each year. The report also points out that people who are HIV-positive can easily be screened for TB and that TB patients can be offered an HIV test.

The African Growth and Opportunity Act. Madeleine Korbel Albright. *US Department of State Dispatch*, v. 9 pp9–11 July 1998.

In an opening statement before the Senate Finance Committee, Washington, D.C., the U.S. secretary of state, Albright, testified on behalf of the African Growth and Opportunity Act. This legislation framed a new U.S. approach to a new Africa by exploring what could be done to build real democracies based on open markets and respect for human rights. It reflected America's policy for placing trade and investment at the forefront of economic relations with Africa and indicated that America is ready to help African nations that help themselves. The bill was designed to encourage African governments to place their economies on a sound financial basis, to allow the emergence of private enterprise, to permit outside investment, and to liberalize trade. It also encouraged African countries to work on such development imperatives as the reduction of poverty, the provision of health care and education, and the fostering of a new generation of entrepreneurs.

Africa: In Search of Solutions. Peter W. Cunningham and Karen L. Ebey-Tessendorf. *World Health*, pp20–1 March/April 1997.

Cunningham and Ebey-Tessendorf propose that the African solution to the problem of supplying primary health care for everyone resides in a fusion of modern and traditional health care. The existence in South Africa and elsewhere of many African professional nurses who are also traditional healers is evidence of this fusion. Many of these women are involved in the antenatal care of pregnant women as traditional healers, but their role is limited as they are not recognized by medical practitioners. All resources, including such women, must be used to the maximum if all of the children in Africa are to benefit from progress in new approaches to antenatal care.

Index